Gastrointestinal Physiology

Gastrointestinal Physiology

Edited by
LEONARD R. JOHNSON, Ph.D.
Thomas A. Gerwin Professor and Chairman
Department of Physiology and Biophysics
University of Tennessee College of Medicine
Memphis, Tennessee

FOURTH EDITION
with **108** *illustrations*

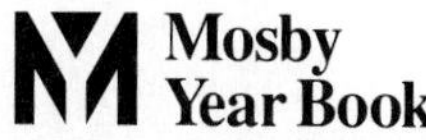

St. Louis Baltimore Boston Chicago London Philadelphia Sydney Toronto

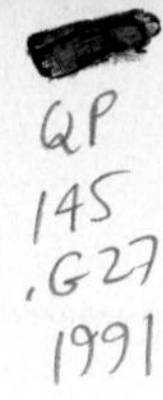

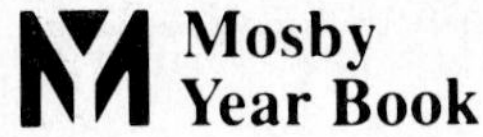

Dedicated to Publishing Excellence

Editor: Kimberly Kist
Assistant Editor: Penny Rudolph
Project Supervisor: Lilliane Anstee
Designer: Elizabeth Fett

FOURTH EDITION

Printed in the United States of America

Mosby-Year Book, Inc.
11830 Westline Industrial Drive, St. Louis, Missouri 63146

Library of Congress Cataloging-in-Publication Data

Gastrointestinal physiology / edited by Leonard R. Johnson. — 4th ed.
p. cm.
Includes bibliographical references.
Includes index.
ISBN 0-8016-5890-X
1. Gastrointestinal system—Physiology. 2. Digestion.
I. Johnson, Leonard R., 1942–
[DNLM: 1. Gastrointestinal System—physiology. WI 102 G2571]
QP145.G27 1991
612.3—dc20
DNLM/DLC
for Library of Congress 90-13415
CIP

UG/DC/DC 9 8 7 6 5 4 3 2 1

Contributors

GILBERT A. CASTRO, Ph.D.
Professor, Department of Physiology and Cell Biology
University of Texas Medical School
Houston, Texas

EUGENE D. JACOBSON, M.D.
Dean, School of Medicine
University of Colorado Health Sciences Center
Denver, Colorado

LEONARD R. JOHNSON, Ph.D.
Thomas A. Gerwin Professor and Chairman
Department of Physiology and Biophysics
University of Tennessee College of Medicine
Memphis, Tennessee

NORMAN W. WEISBRODT, Ph.D.
Professor
Department of Physiology and Cell Biology and Department of Pharmacology
University of Texas Medical School
Houston, Texas

Preface to Fourth Edition

As with any new work, those involved hope that it is better than the previous one. The authors and I feel strongly that this fourth edition is such an improvement. The methods of presentation and philosophy remain the same as in previous editions. However, Dr. Weisbrodt has rewritten the chapters on esophageal and gastric motility to reflect the primary motor functions of those areas, namely swallowing and emptying, respectively. I have also rewritten the chapter on salivary secretion. The material in all chapters has been updated to reflect current knowledge and concepts. Hopefully, we have corrected all errors present in the previous edition without introducing too many new ones.

The entire book is still written by the original authors. I am again indebted to them for their ability to transmit their expertise in a lucid and concise manner. Their contributions arrived on schedule, and anyone who has had the experience of editing a volume realizes how rare this is.

We are all grateful to our own students for pointing out errors and areas of ambiguity. Many colleagues in other medical schools and professional institutions have added their suggestions and criticisms as well. We are thankful for their interest and help, and we hope that anyone having criticisms of this edition or suggestions for improving future editions will transmit them to me or the authors.

Finally, I wish to thank Ms. Doris Parsons for typing many of the chapters and helping with the communications and organizational work that are a necessary part of such a project.

LEONARD R. JOHNSON

Preface to First Edition

The authors of this text have been members of the same medical school department of physiology and have worked together for 4 years to present an integrated and current course in gastrointestinal physiology. This text is, for the most part, a result of this experience and our need for a book on gastrointestinal physiology written and designed for medical students and beginning graduate students.

This material is also meant to serve as a review of modern gastrointestinal physiology for advanced graduate students, interns, residents, and physicians. Important papers and the best available reviews of each subject are included in reference lists at the end of each chapter. Thus the text will serve as a ready departure point for those looking for further information. Current areas of research and controversy are pointed out, although they are not subjected to intense discussion. Every attempt has been made to present the most up-to-date information available and yet organize and synthesize it in an understandable pattern. This was possible because each author is a specialist and currently involved in basic research in the field he has written about.

The first chapter contains a thorough introduction to gastrointestinal endocrinology. As new findings in this field accumulated over the past dozen years, it became apparent that each digestive process is regulated by the combined action of several hormones as well as the nervous system. An overview of this endocrinology is thus essential before one can understand the regulation of a specific process such as gastric acid secretion.

The final chapter covers the entire digestive system and demonstrates how the various processes studied beforehand affect blood flow to and from the gastrointestinal tract. The intervening chapters are arranged in standard fashion and divided into sections on motility, secretion, and digestion and absorption.

At the end of appropriate chapters is a section devoted to clinical tests that are based on the physiological principles discussed in that particular chapter. Throughout each chapter the authors have drawn on clinical material to illustrate important physiological concepts. It is hoped that this will emphasize to the student the importance of understanding normal functions before trying to interpret the abnormal.

The lucid and concise writing style of the authors has made my task as an editor an easy one. In addition, I have had much assistance and advice from the authors regarding content and arrangement. I am grateful to them for their time, concern, and involvement in making this a pleasurable and, what I feel was, a successful task.

LEONARD R. JOHNSON

Contents

1 Regulation Peptides of the Gastrointestinal Tract

Leonard R. Johnson

All gastrointestinal hormones are peptides. It is important, however, to realize that not all peptides found in digestive tract mucosa are hormones. Gastrointestinal tract peptides can be divided into endocrines, paracrines, and neurocrines, depending on the method by which the peptide is delivered to its target site.

Endocrines or hormones are released into the general circulation and reach all tissues (unless excluded from the brain by the blood-brain barrier). Specificity is a property of the target tissue itself. Specific receptors, which recognize and bind the hormone, are present on its target tissues and absent from others. There are four established gastrointestinal hormones; in addition, some gastrointestinal peptides are released from endocrine cells into the blood but have no known physiological function. Conversely, several peptides have been isolated from mucosal tissue and have potent gastrointestinal effects, but no mechanism for their physiological release has been found. Members of these latter two groups are classified as candidate hormones.

Paracrines are released from endocrine cells and diffuse through the extracellular space to their target tissues. Their effects are limited by the short distances necessary for diffusion. Nevertheless, these agents can affect large areas of the digestive tract by virtue of the scattered and abundant distributions of the cells containing them. A paracrine agent also can act on endocrine cells. Thus a paracrine may release or inhibit the release of an endocrine substance, thereby ultimately regulating a process remote from its origin.

Some gastrointestinal peptides are located in nerves and may act as neurocrines or neurotransmitters. A neurocrine is released near its target tissue and needs only to diffuse across a short synaptic gap. Neurocrines conceivably may stimulate or inhibit the release of endocrines or paracrines. Acetylcholine, although not a peptide, is an important neuroregulator in the gastrointestinal tract. One of its actions is to stimulate acid secretion from the gastric parietal cells.

GENERAL CHARACTERISTICS

The gastrointestinal tract is the largest endocrine organ in the body. Its hormones were the first to be discovered. The word "hormone" was coined by W.B. Hardy and used by Starling in 1905 to describe secretin and gastrin and to convey the concept of bloodborne chemical messengers. The gastrointestinal hormones are released from the mucosa of the stomach and small intestine by nervous activity, distention, and chemical stimulation coincident with the intake of food. Released into the portal circulation the gastrointestinal hormones pass through the liver to the heart and back to the digestive system to regulate its movements and secretions. These hormones also regulate the growth of the stomach, small intestine, and pancreas.

Gastrointestinal peptides have many different types of actions. Their effects on water, electrolyte, and enzyme secretion are well known; but they also influence motility, growth, the release of other hormones, as well as intestinal absorption. These processes are summarized and presented in the outline that follows:

1. Water and electrolyte secretion
   a. Stomach
   b. Pancreas
   c. Liver
   d. Gut
2. Enzyme secretion
   a. Stomach
   b. Pancreas
3. Trophic effects
   a. Gastric mucosa
   b. Pancreas
   c. Gut mucosa
4. Endocrine secretion
   a. Gastrointestinal hormones
   b. Insulin
   c. Glucagon
   d. Calcitonin
5. Motility
   a. Stomach
   b. Gut
   c. Sphincters
   d. Gallbladder
6. Intestinal absorption
   a. Water
   b. Electrolytes
   c. Nutrients

Many of these actions overlap; two or more gastrointestinal peptides may affect the same process in the same direction, or they may inhibit each other. Many of the demonstrated actions of these peptides are pharmacological and do not occur under normal circumstances. This chapter will be concerned primarily with the physiological effects of the gastrointestinal peptides.

The actions of the gastrointestinal peptides also may vary in both degree and direction among species. Providing that data are available, the actions discussed in the remainder of this chapter will be those occurring in humans.

DISCOVERY

Four steps are required to establish the existence of a gastrointestinal hormone. First, a physiological event such as a meal must be demonstrated to provide the stimulus to one part of the digestive tract that subsequently alters the activity in another part. Second, the effect must persist after all nervous connections between the two parts of the tract have been severed. Third, from the site of application of the stimulus a substance must be isolated that, when injected into the blood, mimics the effect of the stimulus. Fourth, the substance must be identified chemically and its structure confirmed by synthesis.

Three classic gastrointestinal peptides have achieved full status as hormones. They are secretin, gastrin, and cholecystokinin (CCK).

One recently discovered peptide, gastric inhibitory peptide (GIP), has achieved full hormonal status as the fourth gastrointestinal hormone. There is an extensive list of "candidate hormones," whose significance has not been established. This list includes several chemically defined peptides that have significant actions in physiology or pathology but whose hormonal status has not been proved. These are pancreatic polypeptide, motilin, neurotensin, and substance P. In addition, two known hormones, glucagon and somatostatin, have been identified in gastrointestinal tract mucosa. Their possible function as gastrointestinal hormones is currently being investigated.

Secretin, the first hormone, was discovered in 1902 by Bayliss and Starling and was described as a substance, released from the duodenal mucosa by hydrochloric acid, that stimulated pancreatic bicarbonate and fluid secretion. It was isolated and its amino acid sequence was identified by Jorpes and Mutt in 1966 and synthesized by Bodanszky and coworkers later in the same year.

Edkins discovered gastrin in 1905, stating to the Royal Society that "in the process of the absorption of digested food in the stomach a substance may be separated from the cells of the mucous membrane which, passing into the blood or lymph, later stimulates the secretory cells of the stomach to functional activity." For 43 years investigators were preoccupied by the controversy over the existence of gastrin. The debate intensified when Popielski demonstrated that histamine, a ubiquitous substance present in large quantities throughout the body (including the gastric mucosa), was a powerful gastric secretagogue. In 1938 Komarov demonstrated that gastrin was a polypeptide and was different from histamine. By 1964 Gregory and his colleagues had extracted and isolated hog gastrin. It was synthesized by Kenner and his group in the same year. After 60 years all the criteria for establishing the existence of a gastrointestinal hormone had been satisfied.

In 1928 Ivy and Oldberg described a humoral mechanism for the stimulation of gallbladder contraction initiated by the presence of fat in the intestine. The hormone was named "cholecystokinin" after its primary action. The only controversy involving cholecystokinin is a mild one over nomenclature. In 1943 Harper and Raper described a hormone released from the small intestine that stimulated pancreatic enzyme secretion and accordingly named it pancreozymin. As the purification of these two substances was carried out by Jorpes and Mutt in 1968, it became obvious that both properties resided in the same peptide. For the sake of convenience and because it was the first action described, this hormone was called cholecystokinin.

In 1969 Brown and his co-workers described the purification of a powerful enterogastrone from intestinal mucosa. "Enterogastrone" literally means substance from the intestine *(entero-)* that inhibits *(-one)* the stomach *(gastr-)*. By 1971 this peptide had been purified, isolated, sequenced, and named "gastric inhibitory peptide" after its ability to inhibit gastric secretion. Released from the intestinal mucosa by fat and glucose, GIP also stimulates insulin release. Following the proof that release of insulin was a physiological action of the peptide, GIP became the fourth gastrointestinal hormone. The insulinotropic effect of GIP requires elevated amounts of serum glucose. For this reason, and because it is doubtful whether the inhibitory effects of the peptide on the stomach are physiological, it has been suggested that its name be changed to (G)lucose-dependent (I)nsulinotropic (P)eptide. In either case it is still referred to as GIP.

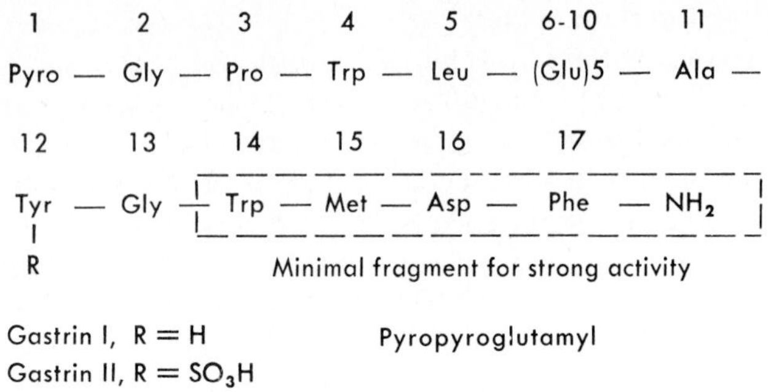

1 2 3 4 5 6-10 11
Pyro — Gly — Pro — Trp — Leu — (Glu)5 — Ala —

12 13 14 15 16 17
Tyr — Gly — Trp — Met — Asp — Phe — NH$_2$
R
Minimal fragment for strong activity

Gastrin I, R = H
Gastrin II, R = SO_3H
Pyropyroglutamyl

Fig. 1-1. Structure of human little gastrin (G 17).

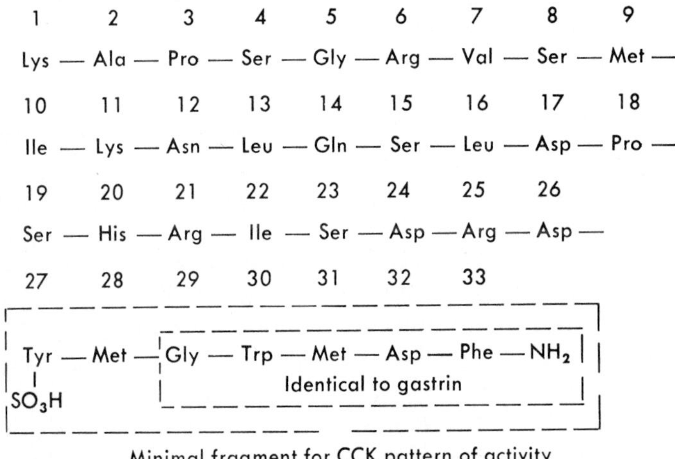

Fig. 1-2. Porcine cholecystokinin.

CHEMISTRY

The gastrointestinal hormones and some related peptides can be divided into two structurally homologous families.

The first consists of gastrin (Fig. 1-1) and CCK (Fig. 1-2). The five carboxy-terminal (C-terminal) amino acids are identical in these two hormones. All the biological activity of gastrin can be reproduced by the four C-terminal amino acids. This tetrapeptide, then, is the minimal fragment of gastrin needed for strong activity and is about one-sixth as active as the whole 17–amino acid molecule. The sixth amino acid from the C-terminus of gastrin is tyrosine, which may or may not be sulfated. When sulfated, the hormone is called *gastrin II.* Both forms occur with equal frequency in nature. The N-terminus of gastrin is pyroglutamyl, and the C-terminus is phenylalamide (Fig. 1-1). Note that the NH_2 group following Phe does not signify that this is the N-terminus but that this C-terminal amino acid is amidated. These alterations in structure protect the molecule from aminopeptidases and carboxypeptidases.

CCK, which has 33 amino acids, contains a sulfated tyrosyl residue in position 7 from the C-terminus. CCK can activate gastrin recep-

	*	1	2	3	4	5	6	7	8	9	10	11	12	13	14	15
Secretin	(27)	His-	Ser-	Asp-	Gly-	Thr-	Phe-	Thr-	Ser-	Glu-	Leu-	Ser-	Arg-	Leu-	Arg-	Asp-
VIP	(28)				Ala-	Val-			Asp-	Asn-	Tyr-	Thr-				Lys-
GIP	(42)	Tyr-	Ala-	Glu-				Ile-		Asp-	Tyr-		Ile-	Ala-	Met-	
Glucagon	(29)			Gln-						Asp-	Tyr-		Lys-	Tyr-	Leu-	

	16	17	18	19	20	21	22	23	24	25	26	27	28	29
Secretin	Ser-	Ala-	Arg-	Leu-	Gln-	Arg-	Leu-	Leu-	Gln-	Gly-	Leu-	Val-NH_2		
VIP	Gln-	Met-	Ala-	Val-	Lys-	Lys-	Tyr-		Asn-	Ser-	Ile-	Leu-	Asn-NH_2	
GIP	Lys-	Ile-		Gln-		Asp-	Phe-	Val-	Asn-	Trp-		Leu-	Ala-	Gln-14 more
Glucagon		Arg-		Ala-		Asp-	Phe-	Val-		Trp-		Met-	Asp-	Thr

*Total amino acid residues
Blank spaces indicate residues identical to those in secretin

Fig. 1-3. Structures of secretin family of peptides.

tors (for example, those for acid secretion); gastrin can activate CCK receptors (for example, those for gallbladder contraction). Each hormone, however, is much more potent at its own receptors than at those of its homologue. CCK is always sulfated in nature, and desulfation produces a peptide with the gastrin pattern of activity. The minimally active fragment for the CCK pattern of activity is therefore the C-terminal heptapeptide. In summary, peptides belonging to the gastrin-CCK family having a tyrosyl residue in position 6 from the C-terminus or in position 7 and unsulfated possess the gastrin pattern of activity—strong stimulation of gastric acid secretion and weak contraction of the gallbladder. Peptides with a sulfated tyrosyl residue in position 7 have cholecystokinetic potency and are weak stimulators of gastric acid secretion. Obviously the tetrapeptide itself and all fragments less than seven amino acids long possess gastrin-like activity.

The second group of peptides is homologous to secretin and includes vasoactive intestinal peptide (VIP), gastric inhibitory peptide (GIP), and glucagon in addition to secretin (Fig. 1-3). Secretin has 27 amino acids, all of which are required for substantial activity. Pancreatic glucagon has 29 amino acids, 14 of which are identical to those of secretin. Glucagon-like immunoreactivity has been isolated from the small intestine, but the significance of this "enteroglucagon" has not been established. Glucagon has no active fragment, and like secretin the whole molecule is required before any activity is observed. There is evidence that secretin exists as a helix; thus the entire amino acid sequence may be necessary to form a tertiary structure with biological activity.

GIP and VIP each have nine amino acids that are identical to those of secretin. Each has many of the same actions as secretin and glucagon. This group of peptides will be discussed in greater detail later in the chapter.

Most peptide hormones are heterogeneous and occur in two or more molecular forms. Gastrin, secretin, and CCK have all been shown to exist in more than one form. Gastrin was originally isolated from hog antral mucosa as a heptadecapeptide (see Fig. 1-1), which is now referred to as "little gastrin" or G 17. It accounts for 90% of antral gastrin. Yalow and Berson demonstrated heterogeneity by showing that the major component of gastrin immunoactivity in the serum was a

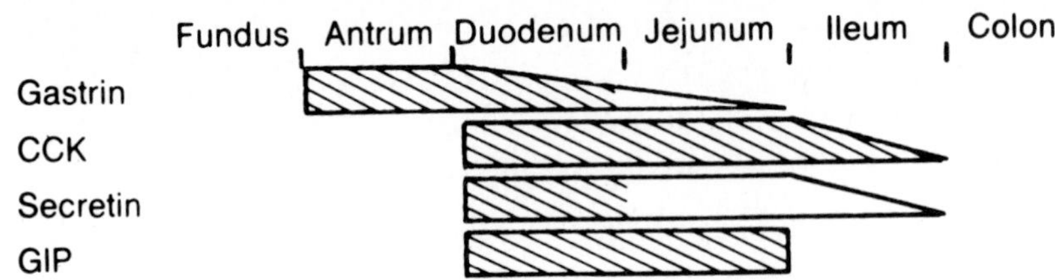

Fig. 1-4. Distribution of the gastrointestinal hormones. Shaded areas indicate where most release occurs under normal conditions.

larger molecule that they called "big gastrin." On isolation big gastrin was found to contain 34 amino acids; hence it is called G 34. Trypsin splits G 34 to yield G 17 plus a heptadecapeptide different from G 17. Therefore G 34 is not simply a dimer of G 17. An additional gastrin molecule (G 14) has been isolated from tissue and contains the C-terminal tetradecapeptide of gastrin. Current evidence indicates that most G 17 is produced from pro G 17 and most G 34 from pro G 34. Thus G 34 is not a necessary intermediate in the production of G 17.

During the interdigestive (basal) state most human serum gastrin is G 34. Unlike that of other species, the duodenal mucosa of humans contains significant amounts of gastrin. This is primarily G 34 and is released in small amounts during the basal state. After a meal a large quantity of antral gastrin, which is primarily G 17, is released and provides most of the stimulus for gastric acid secretion. Smaller amounts of G 34 are released from both the antral and the duodenal mucosa. G 17 and G 34 are equipotent, although the half-life of G 34 is 38 minutes and that of G 17 is about 7 minutes.

DISTRIBUTION AND RELEASE

The gastrointestinal hormones are located in endocrine cells scattered throughout the gastrointestinal mucosa from the stomach through the colon. The cells containing individual hormones are not clumped together but are dispersed among the epithelial cells. The nature of this distribution makes it virtually impossible to surgically remove the source of one of the gastrointestinal hormones and examine the effect of its absence without compromising the digestive function of the animal.

The endocrine cells of the gut are members of a widely distributed system termed "amine precursor uptake decarboxylation" (APUD) cells. These cells are all derived from neuroendocrine-programmed cells originating in the embryonic ectoblast.

The distributions of the individual gastrointestinal hormones are shown in Fig. 1-4. Gastrin is most abundant in antral and duodenal mucosa. Most of its release under physiological conditions is from the antrum. Secretin, cholecystokinin, and GIP are found in the duodenum and jejunum.

Ultrastructurally gastrointestinal endocrine cells have hormone-containing granules concentrated at their bases close to the capillaries. The granules discharge, releasing their hormones in response to a number of events that are either the direct or the indirect result of neural, physical, and chemical stimuli associated with eating a meal and the presence of that meal within the digestive tract. These endocrine cells have microvilli on their apical borders that presumably contain receptors for sampling the luminal contents.

Table 1-1 lists the stimuli that are physiologically important releasers of the gastrointestinal hormones. Gastrin is the only hormone demonstrated to be released directly by neural stimulation. Protein in the form of peptides and single amino acids releases both gastrin and CCK. Fatty acids containing eight or more carbon atoms or their monoglycerides are the most potent stimuli for CCK release. That fat must be broken down into an absorbable form before releasing CCK is evidence that the receptors for release are triggered during the process of absorption. Carbohydrate, the remaining major foodstuff, does not alter the release of gastrin, secretin, or CCK but does stimulate GIP release. GIP also is released by fat and protein. The strongest stimulus for secretin release is hydrogen ion. Secretin is released when the pH in the duodenum falls below 4.5. Secretin also is released by fatty acids. This may be a significant mechanism for secretin release because the concentration of fatty acids in the lumen is often high. CCK also can be released by acid, but, except during hypersecretion of acid, the physiological significance of this mechanism of release has not been established. The purely physical stimulus of distention activates antral receptors, causing gastrin release; for example, inflating a balloon in the antrum will release gastrin. During a meal the pressure of ingested food initiates this response. The magnitude of the response is not as great as originally believed, however, and the contribution that distention makes to the total amount of gastrin released in humans is probably minor. Gastrin also can be released by calcium, decaffeinated coffee, and wine. Pure alcohol in the same concentration as the alcohol in wine does not release gastrin but does stimulate acid secretion.

In addition to releasing secretin, acid exerts an important negative feedback control of gastrin release. Acidification of the antral mucosa below pH 3.5 inhibits gastrin release. Patients with atrophic gastritis, pernicious anemia, or other conditions characterized by the chronic decrease of acid-secreting cells and hyposecretion of acid may have extremely high serum concentrations of gastrin because of the absence of this inhibitory mechanism.

Table 1-1 Releasers of gastrointestinal hormones

	Hormones			
	Gastrin	CCK	Secretin	GIP
Protein	S	S	O	S
Fat	O	S	S−	S
Carbohydrate	O	O	O	S
Acid	I	S−	S	O
Distention	S	O	O	O
Nerve (vagus)	S	O	O	O

S, physiological stimulus for release; S−, of secondary importance; O, no effect; I, inhibits release physiologically.

There are several instances in which hormones alter the release of gastrointestinal peptides. Secretin and glucagon, for example, both inhibit gastrin release. CCK has been shown to stimulate glucagon release, and all four gastrointestinal hormones increase insulin secretion. Elevated serum calcium stimulates both gastrin and CCK release. It is doubtful whether any of these mechanisms, except the release of insulin by GIP, play a role in normal gastrointestinal physiology. Some, however, may become important when circulating levels of hormones or calcium are altered by disease.

ACTIONS AND INTERACTIONS

The effects of pure gastrointestinal hormones have been tested on almost every secretory, motor, and absorptive function of the gastrointestinal tract. Each peptide has some

Table 1-2 Actions of gastrointestinal hormones

Action	Hormones: Gastrin	CCK	Secretin	GIP
Acid secretion	S	S	I	I
Gastric emptying	I	I	I	I
Pancreatic HCO_3^- secretion	S	S	S	O
Pancreatic enzyme secretion	S	S	S	O
Bile HCO_3^- secretion	S	S	S	O
Gallbladder contraction	S	S	S	
Gastric motility	S	S	I	I
Intestinal motility	S	S	I	
Insulin release	S	S	S	S
Mucosal growth	S	S	I	
Pancreatic growth	S	S	S	

S, stimulates; I, inhibits, O, no effect; blank spaces, not yet tested.

action on almost every target tested. Even though large doses of hormone are sometimes necessary to produce an effect, either stimulatory or inhibitory, the fact that receptors for each hormone are present on most target tissues is demonstrated. To indicate the myriad activities possessed by these peptides, many of their actions are summarized in Table 1-2.

The important physiological actions of the gastrointestinal hormones are depicted in Table 1-3. Numerous guidelines have been proposed for determining whether an action is physiological. The action should occur in response to endogenous hormone released by normal stimuli, that is, those present during a meal. In other words, an exogenous dose of hormone should produce the effect in question without elevating serum hormone levels above those produced by a meal. An acceptable guideline for exogenous infusion is the dose that produces 50% of the maximal response (D_{50}) of the primary action of the hormone. The hormone should be administered as a continuous intravenous infusion rather than as a single bolus because the latter produces transient, unphysiologically high serum levels.

The primary action of gastrin is the stimulation of gastric acid secretion. On a molar basis it is 1500 times more potent than histamine. In humans the D_{50} is 1 ng/kg·min. There is considerable debate about the role of gastrin in regulating the tone of the lower esophageal sphincter, with the bulk of evidence indicating no normal role for gastrin in the regulation.

One of the most important and recently discovered actions of gastrointestinal hormones is their trophic activity. Gastrin stimulates synthesis of RNA, protein, and DNA as well as growth of the mucosa of the small intestine, colon, and oxyntic gland area of the stomach. If most endogenous gastrin is removed by antrectomy, these tissues atrophy. Exogenous gastrin prevents the atrophy. Patients with tumors that constantly secrete gastrin exhibit hyperplasia and hypertophy of the acid-secreting portion of the stomach. The trophic effects of gastrin are restricted to gastrointestinal tissues and are counteracted by secretin.

Table 1-3 Important actions of gastrointestinal hormones

Action	Hormones			
	Gastrin	CCK	Secretin	GIP
Acid secretion	S		I	I
Pancreatic HCO_3^- secretion		S	S	
Pancreatic enzyme secretion		S		
Bile HCO_3^- secretion			S	
Gallbladder contraction		S		
Gastric emptying		I		
Insulin release				S
Mucosal growth	S			
Pancreatic growth		S	S	

S, stimulates; I, inhibits.

The trophic action of gastrin is a direct effect that can be demonstrated in tissue culture.

The primary effect of secretin is the stimulation of pancreatic fluid and bicarbonate secretion; one of the primary actions of CCK is the stimulation of pancreatic enzyme secretion. In addition, CCK has a physiologically important interaction in potentiating the primary effect of secretin. Thus CCK greatly increases the pancreatic bicarbonate response to low circulating levels of secretin.

Both CCK and secretin also stimulate the growth of the exocrine pancreas. CCK exerts a stronger effect than does secretin, but the combination of the two hormones produces a potentiated response in rats that is truly remarkable. It is likely that the effects of these two hormones on pancreatic growth are as important as their effects on pancreatic secretion.

In addition to its effects on the pancreas, secretin stimulates biliary secretion of fluid and bicarbonate. This action also is shared by CCK, but secretin is the most potent choleretic of the gastrointesinal hormones. In dogs, secretin is a potent inhibitor of gastrin-stimulated acid secretion. This action, however, probably is not physiologically important in humans. The ability of secretin to inhibit acid secretion may be important in some human diseases, however, and the student should be aware of this action. Secretin has been nicknamed ''nature's antacid,'' for almost all its actions reduce the amount of acid in the duodenum. The only known exception to this general statement is its pepsigogic activity. Secretin is second only to acetylcholine in promoting pepsinogen secretion from the chief cells of the stomach. Under normal circumstances only small amounts of secretin are released, making it doubtful whether secretin stimulates pepsin secretion physiologically.

In addition to its physiologic actions on pancreatic and biliary secretion, CCK regulates gallbladder contraction and gastric emptying. CCK is the most potent regulator of gallbladder contraction of the gastrointestinal peptides. It is approximately 100 times more effective than the gastrin tetrapeptide in contracting the gallbladder. CCK causes significant inhibition of gastric emptying in doses equal to the D_{50} of pancreatic secretion. Gas-

Table 1-4 Candidate hormones

Peptide	Released by	Actions
Pancreatic polypeptide	Protein Fat Glucose	↓Pancreatic HCO_3^- and enzyme secretion
Motilin	?	↑Gastric motility ↑Intestinal motility
Enteroglucagon	Hexose Fat	?

trin also inhibits gastric emptying, but the effective dose is about six times the D_{50} for stimulation of acid secretion by gastrin. This is the type of data that support conclusions that CCK physiologically inhibits gastric emptying and that gastrin does not.

There are several peptides, including secretin and GIP, that are enterogastrones. GIP was originally discovered because of its ability to inhibit gastric acid secretion and may well have been the original enterogastrone described by Ivy and Farrell in 1925. This action has not been established as physiologically significant in the innervated stomach. GIP, however, is a strong stimulator of insulin release and is responsible for the observation that an oral glucose load releases more insulin and is metabolized more rapidly than an equal amount of glucose administered intravenously.

CANDIDATE HORMONES

Earlier in this chapter certain peptides isolated from digestive tract tissue have been mentioned that may, at a later date, qualify as hormones. These often are referred to as "candidate" or "putative" hormones. Many have been proposed, but interest is greatest for those listed in Table 1-4. Enteroglucagon belongs to the secretin family. The others do not appear to be related to either gastrin or secretin.

Pancreatic polypeptide was first identified as a minor impurity in insulin. It was then isolated and found to be a linear peptide with 36 amino acid residues. From a physiological viewpoint the most important action of pancreatic polypeptide is the inhibition of both pancreatic bicarbonate and enzyme secretion, because this effect has the lowest dose requirement. Most constitutents of a meal release pancreatic polypeptide, and the serum levels reached are sufficient to inhibit pancreatic secretion. Because the peak rate of pancreatic secretion during a meal is less than the maximal rate that can be achieved with exogenous stimuli, it is possible that pancreatic polypeptide modulates this response under normal conditions. Before it can be concluded that pancreatic polypeptide is responsible for the physiological inhibition of pancreatic secretion, it must be shown that this actually occurs and that pancreatic polypeptide is the agent involved. The fact that the peptide is located in the pancreas and cannot be removed without also removing its target organ makes this evidence difficult to obtain.

Motilin is a 22–amino acid peptide, isolated from the duodenal mucosa, that stimulates proximal gastrointestinal tract motility. No physiological conditions are known to stimulate its release; however, its concentration in the blood undergoes cyclical fluctua-

Table 1-5 Neurocrines

Peptide	Location	Actions
VIP	Mucosa and muscle of gut	Relaxation of gut smooth muscle
GRP or bombesin	Gastric mucosa	↑Gastrin release
Enkephalins	Mucosa and muscle of gut	↑Smooth muscle tone

tions during fasting. These fluctuations may indicate that its release is under neural control, but this has not been established. The peak blood levels of motilin correspond in time to the beginning of the activity front of the interdigestive migrating myoelectric complex. Exogenous motilin can induce such complexes, indicating that these cycles might be regulated by the release of motilin under normal circumstances.

Enteroglucagon more correctly is termed "glucagon-like immunoactivity," because its presence in intestinal mucosa is detected by radioimmunoassay. After a meal there are appreciable increases in enteroglucagon, but no physiological function for it has been discovered. It is unfortunate that sufficient quantities of enteroglucagon have not been isolated to permit physiological testing.

NEUROCRINES

Originally all gastrointestinal peptides were believed to originate from endocrine cells and therefore to be either hormones or candidate hormones. With the advent of sophisticated immunocytochemical techniques for tissue localization of peptides it became apparent that many were contained within the nerves of the gut.

Numerous peptides have been found in both the brain and the digestive tract mucosa. The first of these to be isolated was substance P, which in the gastrointestinal tract has the property of stimulating intestinal motility and gallbladder contraction. The only other peptide isolated from both the brain and gut and known to have identical structures in both sites is neurotensin. Neurotensin increases blood glucose by stimulating glycogenolysis and glucagon release and inhibiting insulin release. Other peptides have been isolated from one site and identified by radioimmunoassay in the other. These include motilin, CCK, and VIP, which were first isolated from the gut. Enkephalin, somatostatin, and thyrotropin-releasing factor were first isolated from the brain and later found in the gut. Gastrin, VIP, somatostatin, and enkephalin also are present in the nerves of the gut.

There are probably three peptides that function physiologically in the gut as neurocrines. These are listed in Table 1-5. Originally investigators thought VIP was found in gut endocrine cells. It is now known to be localized within the gut exclusively to nerves. It is also the likely physiological mediator of relaxation of gastrointestinal smooth muscle. Smooth muscle is innervated by VIP-containing fibers, and VIP is released during relaxation. VIP relaxes smooth muscle, and VIP antiserum blocks neurally induced relaxation. In addition, there is strong evidence that VIP physiologically mediates relaxation of smooth muscle in blood vessels and thus may be responsible for vasodilation. Besides these effects, VIP has many of the actions of its relatives, secretin and GIP, when injected into the bloodstream. It stimulates pancreatic secretion, inhibits gastric secretion, and stimulates intestinal secretion.

Numerous biologically active peptides have been isolated from amphibian skin and later found to have mammalian counterparts. One of these, called bombesin, after the species of frog from which it was isolated, is a potent releaser of gastrin. The mammalian counterpart of bombesin is gastrin-releasing peptide (GRP) and has been found in the nerves of the gastric mucosa. GRP is released by vagal stimulation and is now considered to mediate the vagal release of gastrin. Luminal protein digestion products also may stimulate gastrin release through a GRP-mediated mechanism.

Two pentapeptides isolated from pig and calf brains activate opiate receptors and are called enkephalins. They are identical except that the carboxy-terminal amino acid is methionine in one and leucine in the other. These compounds are present in nerves within both the smooth muscle and the mucosa of the gastrointestinal tract. Opiate receptors on circular smooth muscle cells mediate contraction; and leu-enkephalin and met-enkephalin cause contraction of the lower esophageal, pyloric, and ileocecal sphincters. The enkephalins probably function physiologically at these sites and also may be an intricate part of the peristaltic mechanism. The effect of opiates on intestinal motility is to slow transit of material through the gut. These peptides also inhibit intestinal secretion. The combination of these actions probably accounts for the effectiveness of opiates in treating diarrhea.

PARACRINES

Paracrines are like hormones in that they are released from endocrine cells. They are similar to neurocrines because they interact with receptors close to the point of their release. The biological significance of an endocrine can be assessed by correlating physiological events with changes in blood levels of the hormone in question. Because the area of release of both paracrines and neurocrines is restricted, there are no comparable methods for proving the biological significance of one of these agents. Current experiments examine the effects of specific pharmacological blockers or antisera directed toward these substances. In vitro perfused organs are also useful in examining paracrine mediators. These systems allow the investigator to collect and assay small volumes of venous perfusate for the agent in question.

One gastrointestinal peptide, somatostatin, appears to function physiologically as a paracrine to inhibit gastrin release. Somatostatin was first isolated from the hypothalamus as a growth hormone release inhibitory factor. It has since been shown to exist throughout the gastric and duodenal mucosa and the pancreas in high concentrations and to inhibit the release of all gut hormones. Recent evidence indicates that somatostatin mediates the inhibition of gastrin release occurring when the antral mucosa is acidified. Somatostatin also directly inhibits acid secretion from the parietal cells. This is also likely to be a physiological action of this peptide.

CLINICAL APPLICATIONS

Non–beta cell tumors of the pancreas or duodenal tumors may produce gastrin and continually release it into the blood. This disease is known as gastrinoma or Zollinger-Ellison syndrome. The tumors are small and difficult to define and resect; and if metastasizing, they grow slowly. Gastrin is released from these tumors at a high spontaneous rate that is not altered by feeding. The hypergastrinemia results in hypersecretion of gastric acid through two mechanisms. First, the trophic action of gastrin leads to increased parietal cell mass and acid secretory capacity. Second, increased serum gastrin levels constantly stimulate secretion from the hyperplastic mucosa. The complications of this disease—fulminant peptic ulceration, diarrhea, steatorrhea, and hypokalemia—are caused by the presence of large amounts of acid in the small bowel. The continual presence of acid in the duodenum overwhelms the neutralizing ability of the pancreas, erodes the mucosa, and produces ulcers. In large amounts gastrin inhibits absorption of fluid and electrolytes by the intestine, thereby adding to the large volumes of fluid (up to 10 L/day) entering the intestine. Increased intestinal transit probably also contributes to the diarrhea. Steatorrhea is produced by inactivation of pancreatic lipase and precipitation of bile salts at low luminal pH. Because the tumors are difficult to resect and the clinical manifestations are caused by hypersecretion of gastric acid, the preferred surgical treatment is removal of the target organ (the stomach). Although gastrin levels remain elevated, total gastrectomy stops the ulceration and diarrhea. This disease also may be treated nonsurgically with some of the powerful new drugs that inhibit acid secretion (see Chapter 8).

The only other clinical condition attributed to the overproduction of a gastrointestinal peptide concerns VIP. Pancreatic cholera or watery diarrhea syndrome is a frequently lethal disease resulting from the secretion of a peptide by a pancreatic islet cell tumor. This peptide is a potent stimulus for intestinal secretion of the fluid and electrolytes that produce the copious diarrhea. VIP has been identified in both tumor tissue and the serum of these patients. Its ability to stimulate cholera-like fluid secretion from the intestine indicates that it is responsible for this disease.

CLINICAL TESTS

Gastrin is the only gastrointestinal hormone for which a reliable radioimmunoassay is readily available for clinical testing. Normal serum gastrin values must be set by each laboratory for its particular assay. If the normal mean serum gastrin concentration is taken as 50 pg/ml, serum gastrin in fasting patients with gastrinoma usually will exceed 200 pg/ml. The degree of overlap between patients with gastrinoma and those with ordinary duodenal ulcer disease means that specific tests are required to diagnose the gastrinoma.

The tests most widely used in the evaluation of hypergastrinemia include stimulation with protein meals, intravenous calcium infusion, and secretin infusion. Patients with Zollinger-Ellison syndrome may not release gastrin in detectable amounts in response to food. This may be due to the low pH of gastric contents caused by ongoing acid secretion stimulated by preexisting high serum gastrin levels. Acid in the antrum inhibits gastrin release, and any gastrin that might be released would be difficult to detect against the already high serum levels.

Gastrinoma patients may have an exaggerated acid secretory response to calcium infusions caused by the release of gastrin from tumor tissue. This test is run by infusing 5 mg of ionizable calcium per kilogram per hour as calcium gluconate for 3 hours while simultaneously measuring acid secretion and collecting blood samples at hourly intervals for gastrin determination. Peak gastrin responses usually are obtained 3 hours after calcium infusion is begun. In most patients with gastrinoma, serum gastrin concentrations will at least double so that the gastrin values will be over 500 pg/ml. Patients with ordinary ulcer disease may show moderate increases in serum gastrin with calcium infusion, but absolute gastrin values after stimulation seldom exceed 200 to 300 pg/ml.

The most specific and easiest test to administer for gastrinoma is secretin injection. Secretin inhibits antral gastrin release and yet stimulates tumor gastrin release in almost all patients with gastrinoma. Secretin (1 U/kg) is given as a rapid intravenous injection and will cause a peak increase in serum gastrin 5 to 10 minutes later. In a patient with definitely increased basal serum gastrin and acid hypersecretion, a doubling of serum gastrin at 5 to 10 minutes strongly indicates the presence of a gastrinoma.

SUGGESTED REFERENCES

Dockray GJ: Physiology of enteric neuropeptides. In Johnson LR, editor: Physiology of the gastrointestinal tract, ed 2, New York, 1987, Raven Press.

Johnson LR: Regulation of gastrointestinal growth. In Johnson LR, editor: Physiology of the gastrointestinal tract, ed 2, New York, 1987, Raven Press.

Makhlouf GM, editor: Handbook of physiology, section 6, The gastrointestinal system, vol 2, Neural and endocrine biology, Bethesda, 1989, American Physiological Society.

Pearse AGE and Takor T: Embryology of the diffuse neuroendocrine system and its relationship to the common peptides, Fed Proc 38:2288-2294, 1979.

Solcia E, Capella C, Buffa R, Usellini L, Fiocca R, and Sessa F: Endocrine cells of the digestive system. In Johnson LR, editor: Physiology of the gastrointestinal tract, ed 2, New York, 1987, Raven Press.

Walsh JH: Gastrointestinal hormones. In Johnson LR, editor: Physiology of the gastrointestinal tract, ed 2, New York, 1987, Raven Press.

Walsh JH and Grossman MI: The Zollinger-Ellison syndrome, Gastroenterology 65:140-165, 1973.

Walsh JH and Grossman MI: Gastrin, N Engl J Med 292:1324-1332; 1337-1384, 1975.

2 Regulation
Nerves and Smooth Muscle

Norman W. Weisbrodt

Digestion and absorption of meals and the maintenance of homeostasis between meals involve the integration of secretory, motility, and absorptive functions of the organs that constitute the gastrointestinal system. This integration is mediated by regulatory systems that monitor events within the body (primarily the gastrointestinal tract) and in the external environment. The information then is processed such that appropriate commands to increase and/or decrease activities of the various organs are given. In all known cases these commands are mediated through the actions of specific chemicals on the target cells of the digestive organs. The manner in which these chemicals reach the target tissues defines the various regulatory systems. In Chapter 1, the endocrine, paracrine, and neurocrine systems were discussed. In this chapter, the role of the nervous system is considered in more detail.

Most secretory, absorptive, and smooth muscle cells in the digestive system possess intrinsic activities that give them a degree of autonomy, which the regulatory systems then modulate. The basic intrinsic properties of each type of secretory and absorptive cell are discussed in separate chapters that deal with the secretion and absorption of specific chemicals. The basic properties and intrinsic activities of the smooth muscle cells will be discussed in this chapter.

ANATOMY OF THE AUTONOMIC NERVOUS SYSTEM

The gastrointestinal tract is innervated by the autonomic nervous system (ANS). It is called the ANS because we normally are not conscious of its activities nor do we exert any willful control over them. The ANS can be divided into the extrinsic nervous system and the intrinsic or enteric nervous system.

The extrinsic nervous system is in turn divided into the parasympathetic and the sympathetic branches (Fig. 2-1). Parasympathetic innervation is supplied primarily by the vagus and pelvic nerves. Long preganglionic axons arise from cell bodies within the medulla of the brain and the sacral region of the spinal cord. These preganglionic nerves enter the various organs of the gastrointestinal tract

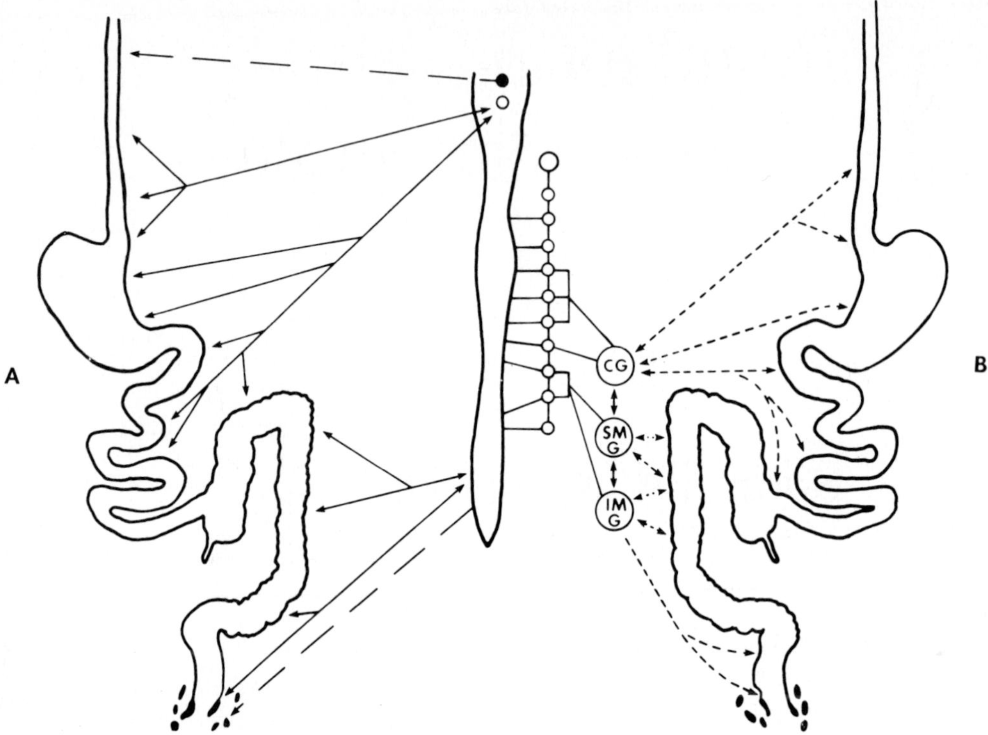

Fig. 2-1. Extrinsic branches of the autonomic nervous system. **A**, Parasympathetic. *Dashed lines* indicate the cholinergic innervation of striated muscle in the esophagus and external anal sphincter. *Solid lines* indicate the afferent and preganglionic efferent innervation of the rest of the gastrointestinal tract. **B**, Sympathetic. *Solid lines* denote the afferent and preganglionic efferent connections between the spinal cord and the prevertebral ganglia (*CG*, celiac; *SMG*, superior mesenteric; *IMG*, inferior mesenteric). *Dashed lines* indicate the afferent and postganglionic efferent innervation.

where they synapse mainly with cells of the enteric nervous system. In addition, these same nerve bundles contain many afferent nerves whose receptors lie within the various tissues of the gut. These nerves project to the brain and spinal cord to provide sensory input for integration.

Sympathetic innervation is supplied by nerves that run between the spinal cord and the prevertebral ganglia and between these ganglia and the organs of the gut. Preganglionic efferent fibers arise within the cord and end in the prevertebral ganglia. Postganglionic fibers from these ganglia then innervate elements of the enteric nervous system. Few fibers end directly on secretory, absorptive, or muscle cells. Afferent fibers also are present within the sympathetic division. These nerves project back to the prevertebral ganglia and/or the spinal cord. Thus an abundance of sensory information is available.

Elements of the intrinsic or enteric nervous system are grouped into several anatomically distinct networks of which the myenteric and submucosal plexuses are the most prominent (Fig. 2-2). These plexuses consist of nerve cell bodies, axons, dendrites, and nerve endings. Processes from the neurons of the plex-

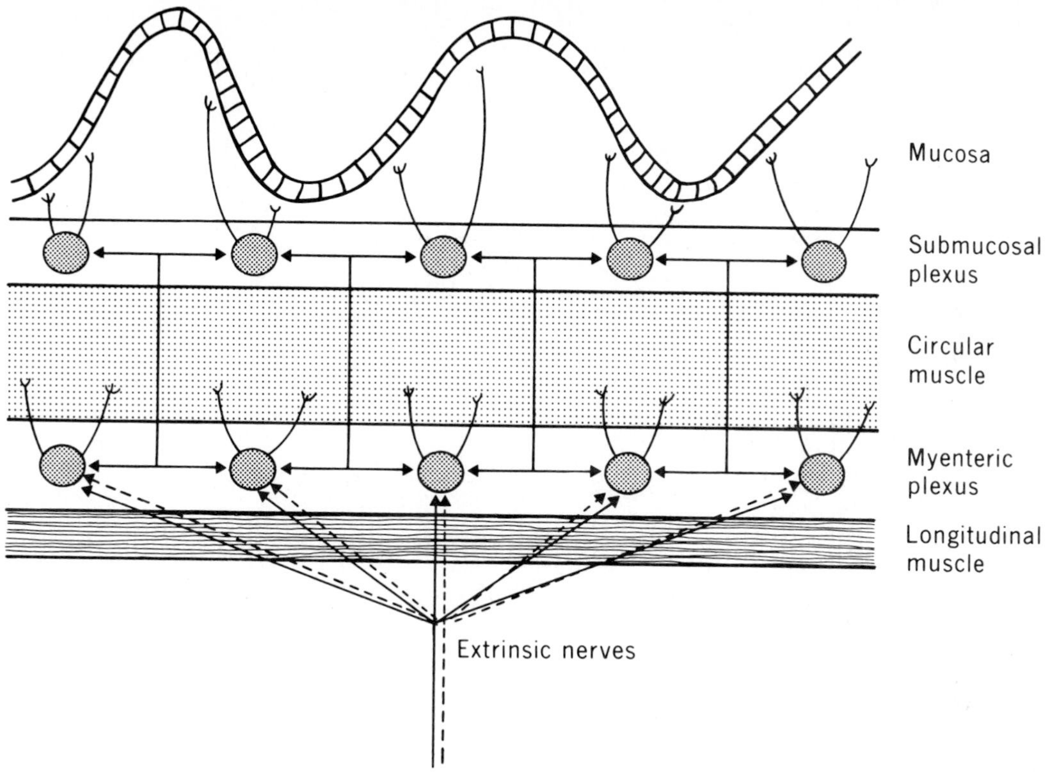

Fig. 2-2. The two main plexuses of the enteric nervous system, myenteric and submucosal, contain numerous cell bodies and processes. Neurons communicate with other neurons in the same plexus and with those in the other plexus. Additionally, plexus neurons communicate with both sympathetic and parasympathetic branches of the extrinsic nerves in the ANS. Plexus neurons receive input from receptors located in the mucosa and muscle layers and supply efferent innervation to those same layers. Thus the enteric nervous system can act autonomously to regulate integrated behavior of the gastrointestinal tract.

uses do not just innervate target cells such as smooth muscle, secretory cells and absorptive cells. They also connect to sensory receptors and interdigitate with processes from other neurons located both inside and outside the plexus. Thus pathways within the enteric nervous system can be multisynaptic, and integration of activities can take place entirely within the enteric nervous system.

There are a large number of chemicals that serve as neurocrines within the ANS. Few of these chemicals have been localized within specific pathways, and few have defined physiological roles. The exceptions to this generalization are acetylcholine and norepinephrine. Most of the preganglionic efferent fibers in both the sympathetic and parasympathetic divisions contain acetylcholine. This transmitter exerts its action on neurons contained within the prevertebral ganglia and the enteric nervous system. Norepinephrine is found in nerve endings of the postganglionic efferent nerves of the sympathetic nervous system. This transmitter also exerts its effects primarily on neurons of the enteric nervous system. Other neurocrines that have been found in the ANS include serotonin, dopamine, and numerous peptides (see Chapter 1). The postulated

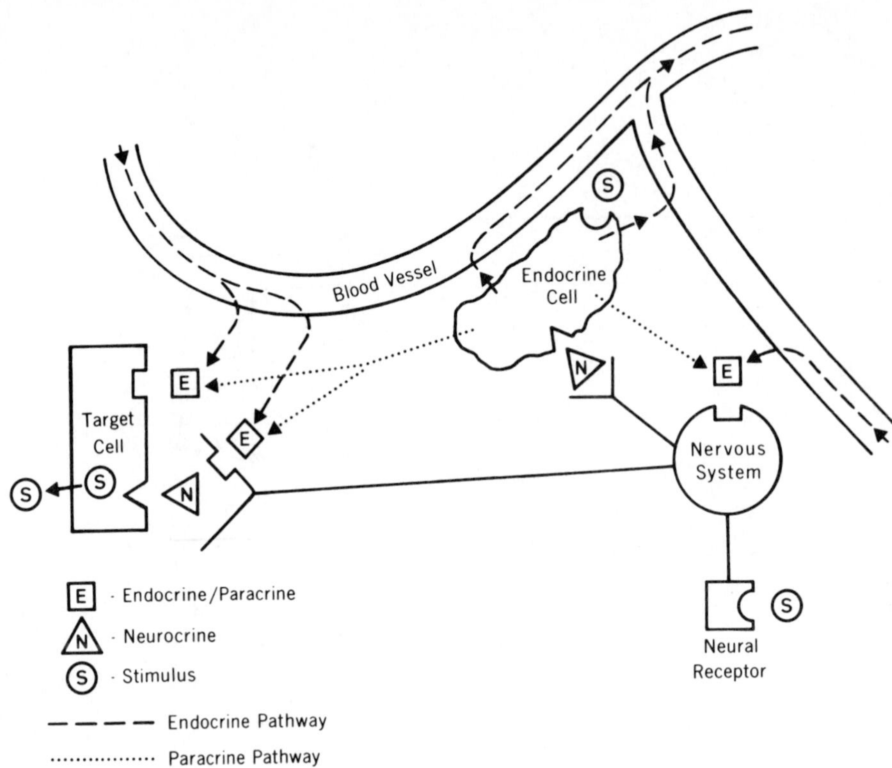

Fig. 2-3. Pathways by which integration of the regulatory systems can occur. Note that most target cells or tissues possess intrinsic activities that are modulated by specific chemicals acting on specific receptors. These chemicals come from nerve endings and endocrine cells. Note also that these same chemicals as well as the products of the target cells can alter activities of the nerves and endocrine cells themselves.

roles for several of these chemicals are stated in the following chapters. For many of these chemicals, however, a specific role is yet to be postulated let alone proven.

NEUROHUMORAL REGULATION OF GASTROINTESTINAL FUNCTION

Although it is convenient to discuss the ANS and the endocrine/paracrine systems separately, it is important to understand that they do not function independently of one another. Rather the regulatory systems interact to control secretion, absorption, and motility. Specific examples of such regulation are given in the following chapters (see Figs. 8-10 and 9-7 for examples). A general scheme of the interaction is depicted in Fig. 2-3. The target cells, be they secretory, absorptive, or smooth muscle cells, have a certain resting output that is modulated by both neurally released and humorally delivered chemicals. These neurocrines, endocrines, and paracrines are released from nerve endings and glandular cells in response to various stimuli that act upon specific receptors. The sources of these stimuli can be either in the environment or within the body. For example, sighting and smelling appetizing food alters many aspects of gastrointestinal function, as does the presence of many food stuffs and products of digestion within the lumen of the stomach and intestine. In many cases the stimuli are the result of the secretory and motor functions of the target cells themselves. Whatever their source, these stimuli initiate signals that are integrated in the neural and endocrine systems in such a way that the output of target cells is modulated appropriately. Thus there are examples of neural activity causing the release of hormones, of hormones modulating neural activity, and of effector cell activity being influenced simultaneously by neural and hormonal activities.

ANATOMY OF THE SMOOTH MUSCLE CELL

The contractile tissue of the gastrointestinal tract is made up of smooth muscle cells except in the pharynx, the orad third of the esophagus, and the external anal sphincter. The smooth muscle cells found in each region of the GI tract exhibit functional and structural differences. These special features are considered in the following chapters. However, certain basic properties are common to all smooth muscle cells. The cells are small compared to skeletal muscle, being some 4 to 10 μm wide and 50 to 200 μm long. A distinguishing feature of these cells is that the contractile elements are not arranged in orderly sarcomeres as in skeletal muscle (Fig. 2-4). Thus the cells have no striations. The contractile proteins, actin and myosin, are present in myofilaments. Actin and tropomyosin constitute the thin filaments, whereas myosin constitutes the thick filaments. Compared to skeletal muscle, smooth muscle contains less myosin, much more actin, and little if any troponin. The apparent ratio of thin to thick filaments in smooth muscles is between 12:1 and 18:1, rather than 2:1, as in skeletal muscle. In addition to the thick and thin filaments, smooth muscle cells contain a third network of filaments that form an internal "skeleton."

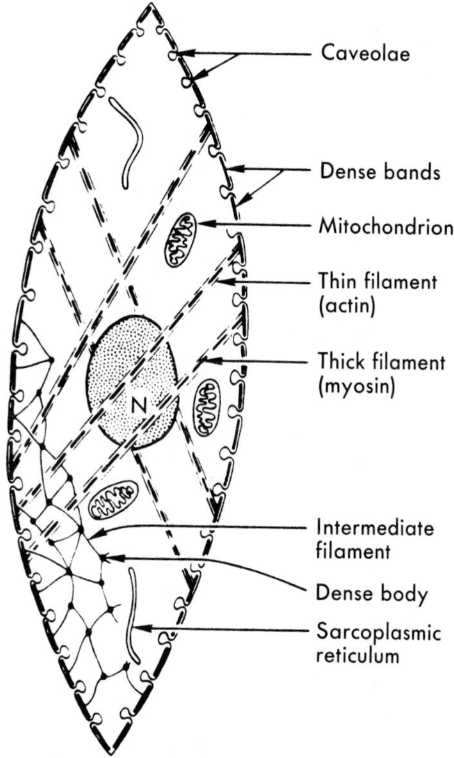

Fig. 2-4. Intracellular structural specializations of a smooth muscle cell. *(Adapted from Schiller LR: In Sleisenger MH and Fordtran JS, editors: Gastrointestinal disease, Philadelphia, 1983, WB Saunders Co.)*

These intermediate filaments, along with their associated dense bodies, may serve as anchor points for the contractile filaments.

Smooth muscle cells of the gastrointestinal tract always occur as elements of the various organs. The cells are arranged in branching bundles or fasciae, surrounded by connective tissue sheets. It is these bundles, organized into muscular coats, that are the effector units.

Smooth muscle tissue of the gut is mostly of the "unitary" type (Fig. 2-5). That is, the individual cells are coupled functionally to one another so that contractions of a bundle of muscle are synchronous. In most tissues this

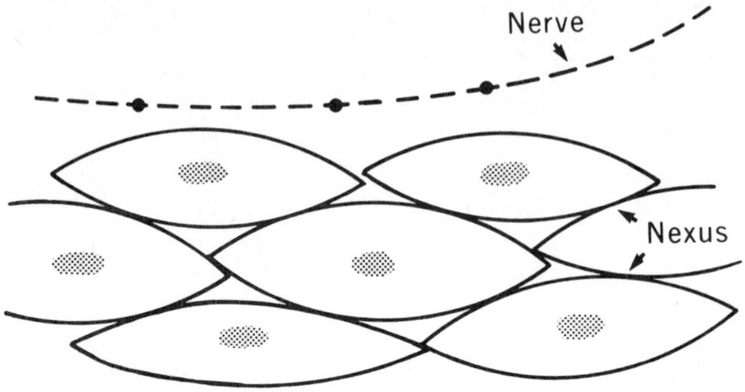

Fig. 2-5. Anatomical features of "unitary" smooth muscle. Neurotransmitter is released from varicosities along the nerve trunk. Other chemicals arrive by endocrine and paracrine routes. The influence of these substances on one muscle cell is then transmitted to other cells by nexuses.

coupling is due to actual fusion of apposing membranes in the form of gap junctions or nexuses. These junctions serve as areas of low resistance for the spread of excitation from one cell to another. Not every smooth muscle cell is innervated. Nerve axons enter the muscle bundles and release neurotransmitters from swellings along their length. These swellings are usually some distance from the muscle cells so that no discrete neuromuscular junctions exist. Thus the neurotransmitters probably act only on a few of the cells. The influence of the transmitters then must be communicated from one smooth muscle cell to the next.

SMOOTH MUSCLE CONTRACTION

There is a remarkable heterogeneity in the time course of contractions among smooth muscles in the gastrointestinal tract. Some muscles, such as those found in the body of the esophagus, the small bowel, and the gastric antrum, contract and relax in a matter of seconds. Thus they are said to contract "phasically." Other smooth muscles such as those found in the lower esophageal sphincter, the orad stomach, and the ileocecal and internal anal sphincters show sustained contractions that last from minutes to hours. These muscles exhibit what are called "tonic" contractions. As discussed in the following chapters the type of contraction, whether phasic or tonic, is governed by the smooth muscle cells themselves. It does not depend upon neural or hormonal input. Neurocrines, endocrines, and paracrines are important in that they modulate the basic contractile activity, causing the amplitude of the contractions of phasic muscles to vary and the tone of the tonic muscles to increase or decrease.

As in other muscle cells, contractile activity is modulated by the levels of free intracellular calcium. At low levels ($<10^{-7}$ M) of calcium, interaction of the contractile proteins does not occur. At higher levels of calcium, proteins interact and contractions occur.

The prevailing theory for the regulation of contraction is that the calcium combines with the calcium-binding protein, calmodulin, and the complex activates a protein kinase that brings about the specific phosphorylation of one of the components of myosin (Fig. 2-6). Myosin in its phosphorylated form then interacts with actin to cause contraction, which is fueled by the splitting of ATP. When the intracellular levels of calcium fall the myosin is dephosphorylated by a specific phosphatase. This brings about a cessation of the interaction

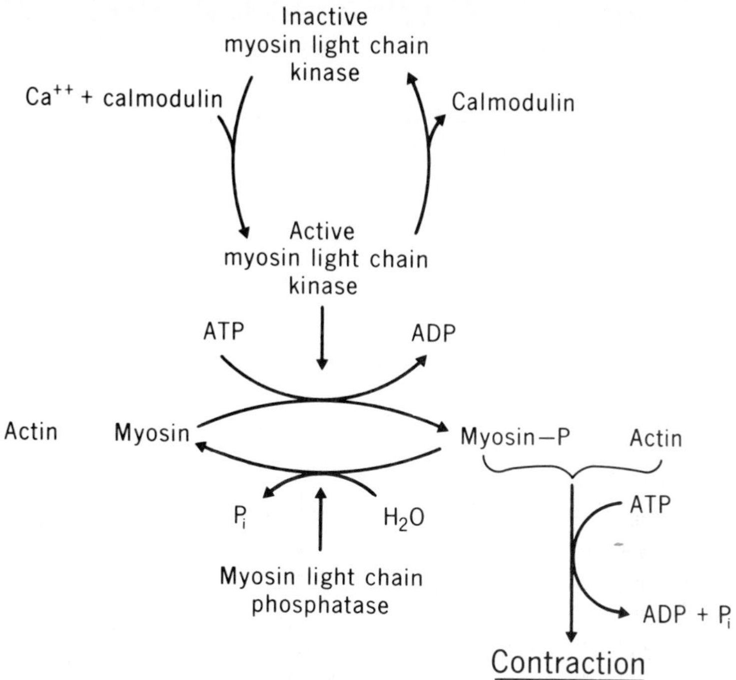

Fig. 2-6. Biochemical events in smooth muscle contraction. An increase in the levels of Ca^{++} activates an enzyme (myosin light chain kinase), which phosphorylates myosin. Phosphorylated myosin *(myosin-P)* interacts with actin to cause muscle contraction. When Ca^{++} levels fall the kinase becomes inactive and the activity of myosin light chain phosphatase dominates. Myosin-P is dephosphorylated and the muscle relaxes.

between the contractile proteins, and causes muscle relaxation.

The exact source of the calcium that participates in the contractile process is not certain. In most gastrointestinal smooth muscles the calcium must enter the cells from the extracellular fluid or from pools of calcium that are bound tightly to the smooth muscle cell membranes or contained in caveoli (Fig. 2-4). Influx of calcium from these sites is regulated by permeability changes of the membrane, which also cause characteristic electrical activities (see below). Some calcium is sequestered in intracellular structures called the sarcoplasmic reticulum (see Fig. 2-4). Although this reticulum is not highly developed in smooth muscle cells, significant amounts of calcium are stored there and are released in response to electrical events of the plasma membrane and to agonist-induced increases in inositol trisphosphate. In addition to these sources for calcium, mechanisms also exist for the expulsion of calcium from the cells and for reuptake into the sarcoplasmic reticulum.

Increases in free intracellular calcium are related to the electrical activities of the smooth muscle cell membranes. In phasically active muscle, calcium enters the cell by way of voltage-dependent calcium channels. When these are activated, rapid transients in membrane potential called *action* or *spike* potentials occur (Fig. 5-6). In many phasic muscles these spike potentials do not arise from a stable resting membrane potential. Rather they are superimposed on relatively slow (3 to 12 cycles/min) but regular oscillations in membrane potential. These potential changes, called "slow waves," do not in themselves cause significant contractions. However, they set the timing for spike potentials to occur, because spikes are seen only during the peak depolarization of the slow wave. The genesis of slow waves has not been elucidated. One theory holds that they are caused by cyclical activity of an electrogenic Na^+ pump.

Both slow waves and spike potentials are inherent in the smooth muscle cells themselves. Slow waves are extremely regular and are influenced only minimally by neural or hormonal activities. They are influenced by body temperature and metabolic activity. The higher the activity, the higher the frequency of slow waves. On the other hand the occurrence of spike potentials depends heavily upon neural and hormonal activities.

In summary, an excitatory endocrine, paracrine, or neurocrine will act on a receptor on the smooth muscle cell membrane to induce spike potentials in those cells and in adjacent cells that are coupled to those cells. The spike potentials lead to an increase in intercellular free Ca^{++} levels. The Ca^{++} then acts via myosin light chain kinase to induce contraction. An inhibitory mediator will act with its receptor on that same membrane. In this case, however, the response will be an inhibition of spike potentials and/or a hyperpolarization of the cell membrane. This results in a decrease in intracellular free Ca^{++} and subsequent relaxation. It is the interplay of these excitatory and inhibitory mediators on the basal activity of the muscle that determines the motility functions of the various organs of the gut.

SUGGESTED REFERENCES

Costa M, Furness JB, and Llewellyn-Smith IJ: Histochemistry of the enteric nervous system. In Johnson LR, editor: Physiology of the gastrointestinal tract, ed 2, New York, 1987, Raven Press.

Gabella G: Structure of muscles and nerves in the gastrointestinal tract. In Johnson LR, editor: Physiology of the gastrointestinal tract, ed 2, New York, 1987, Raven Press.

Murphy RA: Contraction of muscle cells. In Berne RM and Levy MN, editors: Physiology, St Louis, 1988, The CV Mosby Co.

Murphy RA: Muscle as a tissue. In Berne RM and Levy MN, editors: Physiology, St Louis, 1988, The CV Mosby Co.

Roman C and Gonella J: Extrinsic control of digestive tract motility. In Johnson LR, editor: Physiology of the gastrointestinal tract, ed 2, New York, 1987, Raven Press.

Wood JD: Electrical and synaptic behavior of enteric neurons. In Schultz SG, Wood JD, and Rauner BB, editors: Handbook of physiology: the gastrointestinal system, vol 4, Bethesda, 1989, American Physiological Society.

3 Swallowing

Norman W. Weisbrodt

The movement of food through the gastrointestinal tract begins with its oral ingestion. Liquids, unless they are to be savored, are swallowed immediately. Solid particles usually are first reduced in size and mixed with saliva through the process of chewing. Little digestion or absorption takes place during swallowing. It is almost purely a motility function, transporting material into the stomach in a matter of seconds.

The process of swallowing involves the integrated contractile activities of the oral cavity, pharynx, esophagus, and orad portion of the stomach. It is initiated by propulsion of material into the oropharynx primarily by movements of the tongue. The portion to be swallowed is separated from other material in the mouth so it lies in a chamber created by placing the tip of the tongue against the hard palate (Fig. 3-1, *A*). It is propelled by elevation and retraction of the tongue against the palate. As the material passes into the oropharynx the nasopharynx is closed by movement of the soft palate and contraction of the superior constrictor muscles of the pharynx (Fig. 3-1, *B*). Simultaneously, respiration is inhibited and contraction of the laryngeal muscles closes the glottis and raises the larynx. The bolus is propelled through the pharynx by a peristaltic contraction that begins in the superior constrictor and progresses through the middle and inferior constrictor muscles of the pharynx (Fig. 3-1, *C*). These contractions, along with relaxation of the upper esophageal sphincter, propel the bolus into the esophagus (Fig. 3-1, *D*).

The oral and pharyngeal phases of swallowing are extremely rapid, taking less than 1 second. Swallowing can be initiated voluntarily. Once initiated, however, it proceeds as a coordinated involuntary reflex. Coordination is central in origin, and an area within the reticular formation of the brainstem has been identified as the "swallowing center." Afferent impulses from the pharynx are directed toward this center, which serves to coordinate activity of other areas of the brain such as the nuclei of the trigeminal, facial, and hypoglossal nerves, as well as the nucleus ambiguous (Fig. 3-2). Efferent impulses from the center are

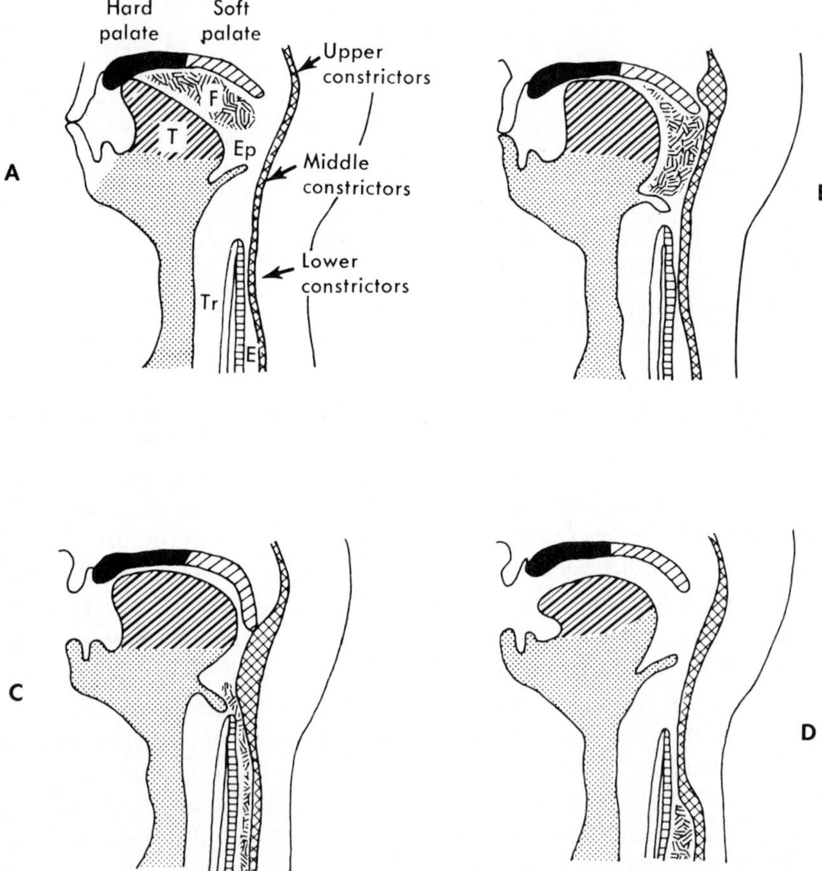

Fig. 3-1. Oral and pharyngeal events during swallowing. **A**, The bolus (*F*) to be swallowed is propelled into the pharynx by placement of the tongue (*T*) on the roof of the hard palate. **B**, Further propulsion is caused by movement of the more distal regions of the tongue against the palate. Contraction of the upper constrictors of the pharynx and movement of the soft palate separate the oropharynx from the nasopharynx. **C**, Propulsion through the upper esophageal sphincter is accomplished by contraction of the middle and lower constrictors of the pharynx and by relaxation of the cricopharyngeal muscle. Upward movement of the glottis and downward movement of the epiglottis (*Ep*) seal off the trachea (*Tr*). **D**, The bolus is now in the esophagus (*E*) and is propelled into the stomach by a peristaltic contraction.

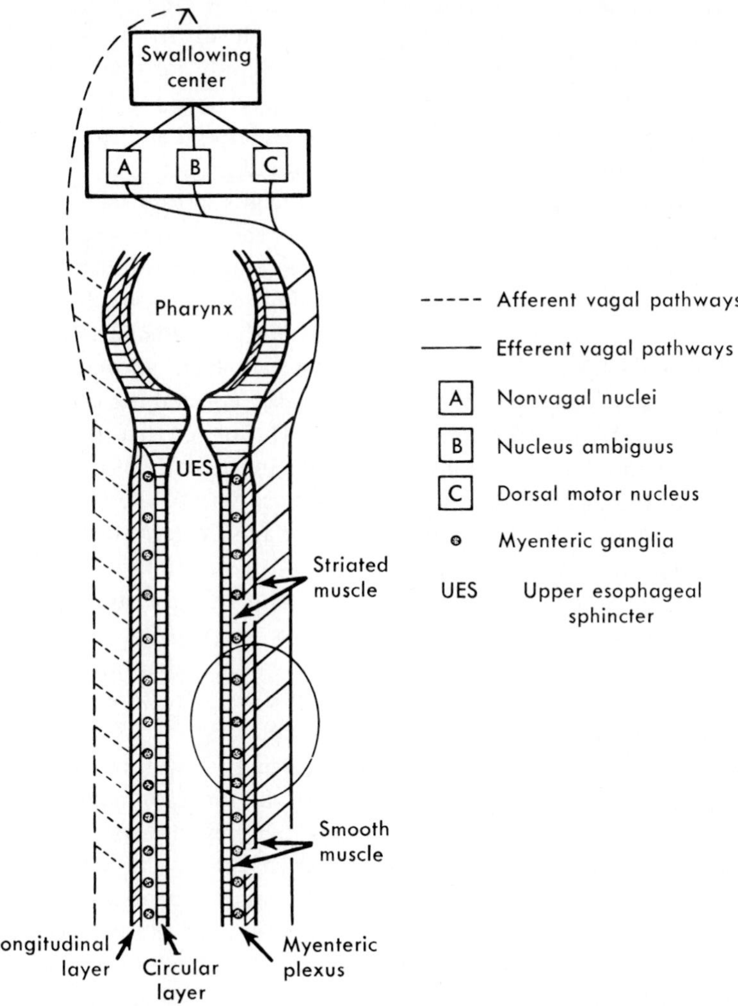

Fig. 3-2. Control of pharyngeal and esophageal peristalsis. Sensory input from the pharynx activates an area in the medulla (the "swallowing center"). This center serves to coordinate activation of the vagal nuclei with other centers such as the respiratory centers. Muscles of the pharynx and striated areas of the esophagus are activated via the center by the nucleus ambiguus. Areas of the smooth muscle are activated via the dorsal motor nucleus. Peristalsis is caused by sequential activation of the muscles of the pharynx and esophagus by sequential neural impulses from the center. The area enclosed within the circle is shown in more detail in Fig. 3-4.

distributed to the pharynx via nerves from the nucleus ambiguous. The impulses appear to be sequential so the pharyngeal musculature is activated in a proximal-to-distal manner. This sequencing accounts for the peristaltic nature of the pharyngeal contractions. The center also appears to interact with other areas of the brain involved with respiration and speech. Ablation of the swallowing center produces loss of the pharyngeal component of swallowing.

ESOPHAGEAL PERISTALSIS

The esophagus propels material from the pharynx to the stomach. This propulsion is accomplished by coordinated contractions of the muscular layers of the body of the esophagus. Because a large segment of the esophagus is located in the thorax, where the pressure is lower than in the pharynx and stomach, the esophagus also must withstand entry of air and gastric contents. The barrier functions of the esophagus are accomplished by the presence of sphincters at each end of the organ.

Anatomically the esophageal muscle is arranged in two layers: an inner layer with the muscle fibers organized in a circular axis, and an outer layer with the fibers organized in a longitudinal axis. The upper esophageal sphincter consists of a thickening of the circular muscle and can be identified anatomically as the cricopharyngeal muscle. This muscle, like the musculature of the proximal third of the esophageal body, is striated. The distal third of the esophagus is composed of smooth muscle; although the terminal 1 to 2 cm of the musculature acts as a sphincter, no separate sphincter muscle can be identified anatomically. The middle third of the body of the esophagus is composed of a mixture of muscle types with a descending transition from striated to smooth fibers.

The events that occur in the esophagus between and during swallowing often are monitored by placing pressure-sensing devices at various levels in the esophageal lumen. Such devices indicate that between swallows both the upper and the lower esophageal sphincters are closed and the body of the esophagus is flaccid (Fig. 3-3, *A*). At the upper end of the esophagus a zone of 1 to 2 cm is detected where the pressure exceeds that on either side of the zone by as much as 60 mm Hg. A zone of elevated pressure also is found at the lower end of the esophagus. The length of this zone may vary from several millimeters to a few centimeters, and the pressure may be 20 to 40 mm Hg higher than that on either side. Pressures in the body of the esophagus are similar to those within the body cavity in which the esophagus lies. In the thorax the pressure varies with respiration, dropping with inspiration and rising with expiration. These fluctuations in pressure with respiration reverse below the diaphragm, and intraluminal esophageal pressure reflects intraabdominal pressure.

During a swallow the sphincters and the body of the esophagus act in a coordinated manner (Fig. 3-3, *B*). Shortly before the distal pharyngeal muscles contract the upper esophageal sphincter opens. Once the bolus passes the sphincter closes and assumes its resting tone. The body of the esophagus undergoes a peristaltic contraction. This contraction begins just below the upper esophageal sphincter and occurs sequentially, giving the appearance of a contractile wave moving toward the stomach. After the contractile sequence passes the esophageal muscle becomes flaccid again. Shortly before the peristaltic contraction reaches the lower esophageal sphincter (LES), the sphincter relaxes. After passage of the bolus the sphincter contracts back to its resting level. Unlike the extremely rapid events in the pharynx, esophageal peristalsis is slow. The peristaltic contraction moves down the

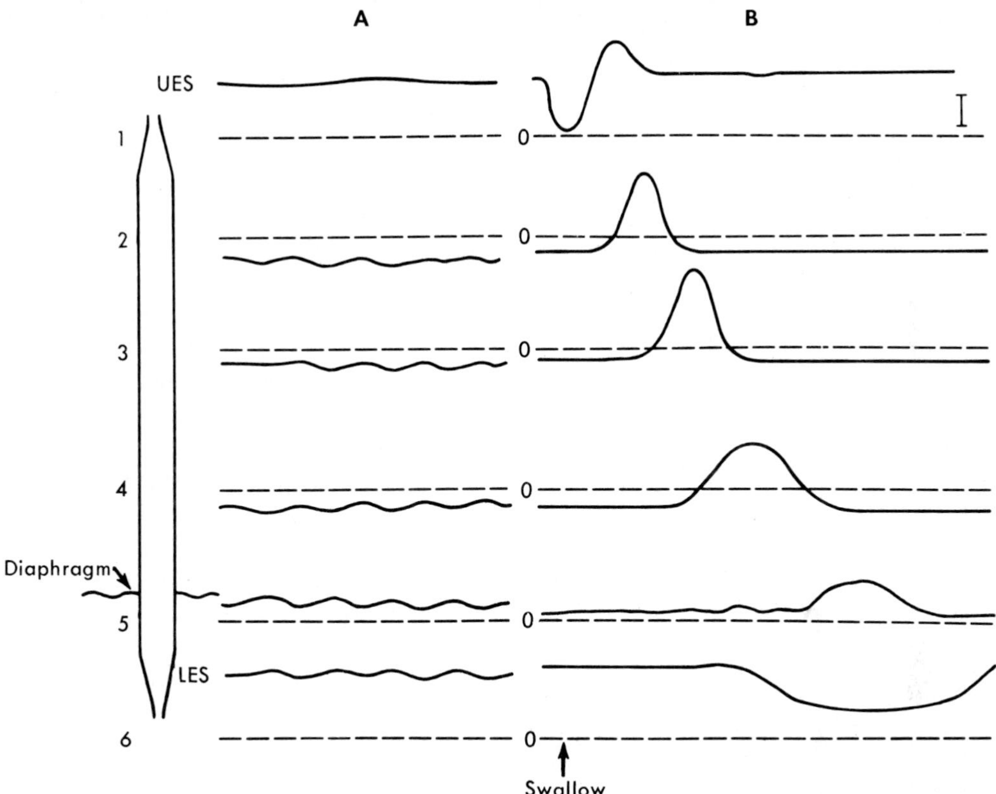

Fig. 3-3. Manometric recording of esophageal contraction. Intraluminal pressures from the upper esophageal sphincter (*UES*), four areas of the esophagus, and the lower esophageal sphincter (*LES*) are shown. **A**, Between swallows both the upper and the lower sphincters are closed, as indicated by the greater than atmospheric pressures recorded there. Pressures in the body of the esophagus reflect intrathoracic or intraabdominal pressures. **B**, On swallowing the upper sphincter relaxes before passage of the bolus. After bolus passage it contracts, to be followed by a peristaltic contraction in the body of the esophagus. To allow passage of the bolus into the stomach, the lower sphincter relaxes before the peristaltic contraction reaches it.

esophagus at velocities ranging from 2 to 6 cm/sec, and may take 10 seconds to reach the lower end of the esophagus.

When esophageal peristalsis is preceded by a pharyngeal phase, it is called "primary peristalsis." Esophageal contractions, however, can occur in the absence of both oral and pharyngeal phases. This is called "secondary peristalsis" and is elicited when the esophagus is distended. Secondary peristalsis occurs if the primary contraction fails to empty the esophagus or when gastric contents reflux into the esophagus. Initiation of secondary peristaltic contractions is involuntary and normally is not sensed.

The effect of esophageal peristalsis on bolus transport depends upon the physical properties of the bolus. If a person in an upright position swallows a liquid bolus, it actually reaches the stomach several seconds before the peristaltic contraction. Thus, although both sphincters must relax to allow transport

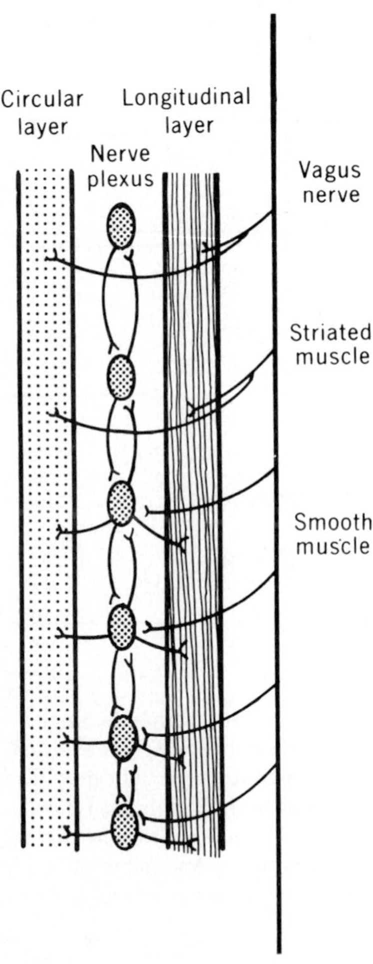

Fig. 3-4. Efferent innervation of the body of the esophagus. Special visceral somatic fibers directly innervate the striated muscle fibers of the circular and longitudinal muscle layers. Preganglionic fibers from the vagus innervate the ganglion cells of the intrinsic plexus. Fibers from the ganglion cells then innervate the smooth muscle cells of both layers. In addition, the ganglion cells have neural connections with one another.

of all materials, esophageal peristalsis is not always necessary. For most swallowed material, peristaltic contractions are essential for progression to the stomach, and repetitive secondary contractions often are required to sweep the bolus completely into the stomach.

Control of esophageal peristalsis is complex and not understood fully. Closure of the upper esophageal sphincter is maintained by the normal elasticity of the sphincteric structures as well as the active contraction of the cricopharyngeal muscle. Relaxation of the upper esophageal sphincter is coordinated with contraction of the pharyngeal musculature. As the larynx rises during the pharyngeal component of swallowing, the cricopharyngeal area is displaced. This displacement, along with relaxation of the cricopharyngeal muscle, allows the sphincter to open. Relaxation of the cricopharyngeal muscle is brought about by a suppression of nerve impulses from the swallowing center caused by the activity of the nucleus ambiguous.

Contractions of the body of the esophagus are coordinated by both central and peripheral mechanisms. The body of the esophagus is innervated primarily by the vagus nerves. These nerves are partly of the somatic motor type, arising from the nucleus ambiguous, and partly of the visceral motor type, arising from the dorsal motor nucleus. The somatic motor nerves synapse directly with striated muscle fibers of the esophagus (Fig. 3-4). The visceral motor nerves supposedly synapse directly not with the smooth muscle cells but with nerve cell bodies that lie between the longitudinal and circular muscle layers. These local nerves, in turn, innervate the smooth muscle cells as well as communicate with one another along the length of the esophagus.

Central control originates within the swallowing center, which sends a series of sequential impulses to progressively more distal segments of the esophagus. This sequential activation results in a peristaltic contraction. The central nervous system does not control peristalsis totally, however. In smooth muscle areas of the esophagus, peristalsis can occur after bilateral cervical vagotomy. Furthermore, peristalsis can be induced in excised esophagi that have been placed in an organ bath. In these instances, peristalsis must be coordinated by the intrinsic nerve plexuses or the smooth muscle cells themselves.

Esophageal peristalsis, also altered by afferent nerve activity, is initated by both the act of swallowing and distention of the esophagus (as indicated by the presence of secondary peristalsis). Besides initiating secondary peristalsis, afferent input may affect the intensity of esophageal muscle contraction. Variation in the size of the bolus being swallowed leads to a variation in the amplitude of esophageal contraction. Indeed, afferent stimulation appears so important that a peristaltic sequence may not occur unless a bolus is swallowed and elicits afferent stimulation. On the other hand, intense afferent stimulation such as the distention of a balloon in the body of the esophagus can inhibit the progression of the peristaltic contraction past the balloon.

Activity of the lower esophageal sphincter is regulated by the intrinsic properties of the smooth muscle fibers as well as by neural and humoral influences. Smooth muscle from this area of the esophagus responds to passive stretching by contracting to oppose the stretch. This response does not depend on nervous activity. Thus the basic tone of the lower esophageal sphincter may be totally myogenic. Nevertheless, this tone is under a number of neural and humoral influences. Resting tone is increased by agents that mimic acetylcholine and by the gastrointestinal hormone gastrin. Sphincteric tone is decreased by agents such as isoproterenol and prostaglandin E_1.

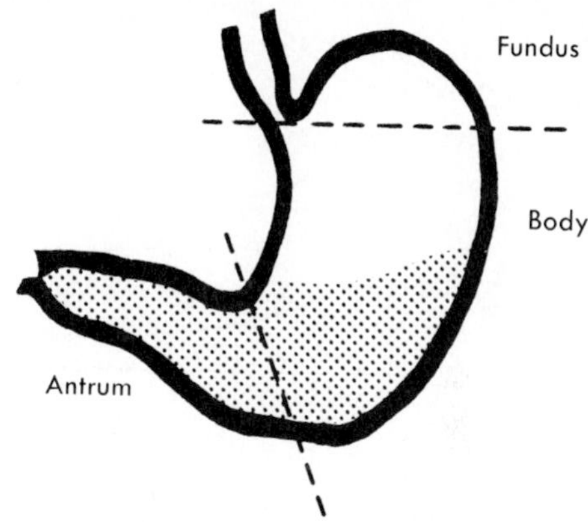

Fig. 3-5. Divisions of the stomach. For discussions of secretion the stomach usually is divided into fundus, body, and antrum. For discussions of motility it can be divided into an orad area and a caudad area. *Stippling* denotes the approximate extent of the caudad area.

Although sphincter tone can be altered by various humoral agents, relaxation during swallowing is mediated neurally. Stimulation of the vagus nerves results in an abrupt fall in sphincter tone. The neurochemical basis for this response is not known, although a role for VIP has been proposed.

RECEPTIVE RELAXATION OF THE STOMACH

Swallowing also involves a region of the stomach. In terms of motile functions the stomach can be divided into two major areas: the orad portion, which consists of the fundus and a portion of the body, and the caudad portion, which consists of the distal body and the antrum (Fig. 3-5). These two regions have markedly different patterns of motility that are responsible, in part, for two major functions: accommodation of ingested material during swallowing, and regulation of gastric emptying. Accommodation is primarily attributable

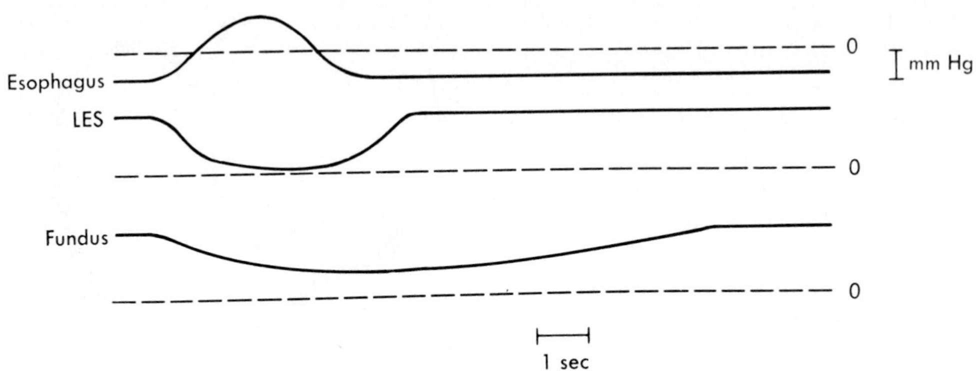

Fig. 3-6. Pressures within the orad region *(Fundus)* of the stomach, the lower esophageal sphincter (*LES*), and the body of the esophagus. Resting pressure within the fundus is slightly above atmospheric pressure. With swallowing the fundus relaxes before arrival of the bolus. After passage of the bolus into the stomach, fundic pressure returns to approximately the previous level.

to activities of the orad region, while both regions are involved in the regulation of gastric emptying (see Chapter 4).

During a swallow the orad region of the stomach relaxes at about the same time as the LES. Intraluminal pressures in both regions fall before the arrival of the swallowed bolus because of the active relaxation of the smooth muscle in both regions (Fig. 3-6). After passage of the bolus the pressure in the stomach returns to approximately what it was before the swallow. This process has been termed "receptive relaxation." Because relaxation happens with each swallow, large volumes can be accommodated with a minimal rise in intragastric pressure. For example, the human stomach can accept 1600 ml of air with a rise in pressure of no more than 10 mm Hg.

Receptive relaxation is mediated by a nervous reflex that has its afferent and efferent pathways in the vagus nerve. If this nerve is transected, receptive relaxation is impaired and the stomach becomes less distensible. The neurotransmitter that mediates receptive relaxation is unknown.

CLINICAL APPLICATIONS

Contractions of pharyngeal muscle are controlled solely by extrinsic nerves. Therefore certain neurological diseases (such as cerebrovascular accident) can have an adverse effect on this phase of swallowing. Aspiration often occurs following a neurological lesion because propulsion in the pharynx and upper esophageal sphincter is no longer coordinated. A similar clinical picture can be seen in diseases that affect striated muscle or the myoneural junction.

Diseases affecting the smooth muscle portion of the esophagus predictably cause abnormalities in peristalsis and in the tone of the lower esophageal sphincter. In one disease, achalasia, the lower esophageal sphincter often fails to relax completely with swallowing. This may be coupled with loss of peristalsis in the esophageal body (complete absence of contractions or appearance of simultaneous rather than sequential contractions), resulting in impaired transit. These patients have considerable difficulty swallowing, often aspirate retained esophageal content, and may become severely malnourished. In another disease, diffuse esophageal spasm, simultaneous contraction of long duration and high amplitude can occur. Affected individuals have difficulty swallowing and may complain of chest pain. Although not always symptomatic, abnormalities in the esophageal component of swallowing can occur as part of a variety of systemic diseases. Examples are diabetes mellitus, chronic alcoholism, and scleroderma.

Motor dysfunction also can play an important supporting role in the pathogenesis of other esophageal diseases. One common example is acid injury to the esophageal mucosa, which results from reflux of gastric contents. Often underlying this problem are abnormally low resting pressures in the lower esophageal sphincter and poor or ineffective secondary peristalsis in the esophageal body. The causes of these motor abnormalities are unknown.

CLINICAL TESTS

Swallowing is assessed clinically by x-ray examination with barium and by esophageal manometry.

In the x-ray study the patient swallows a bolus of liquid barium sulfate. This material is radiopaque and thus can be observed fluoroscopically and recorded on the x-ray film as it traverses the esophagus, providing a qualitative description thereby of motor events in both the pharynx and the esophagus.

If a more detailed description of events is required or there is a suspicion of motor disorders such as those just described, esophageal manometry is often useful. Pressures are recorded at various loci by catheters passed through the nose or mouth into the esophagus. While readings are being obtained at various points simultaneously, the patient is given small sips of water to swallow. The recorded pressure changes created by esophageal contractions and variations in sphincter tension can provide a quantitative description of events that occur during swallowing.

SUGGESTED REFERENCES

Christensen J: Motor functions of the pharynx and esophagus. In Johnson LR, editor: Physiology of the gastrointestinal tract, ed 2, New York, 1987, Raven Press.

Goyal RK and Paterson WG: Esophageal motility. In Schultz SG, Wood JD, and Rauner BB, editors: Handbook of physiology: the gastrointestinal system, vol 1, Bethesda, 1989, American Physiological Society.

Roman C and Gonella J: Extrinsic control of digestive tract motility. In Johnson LR, editor: Physiology of the gastrointestinal tract, ed 2, New York, 1987, Raven Press.

4 Gastric Emptying

Norman W. Weisbrodt

Ingested food and drink are stored temporarily in the stomach, where they are mixed with gastric juice and churned to reduce the size of any solid particles. As this is occurring, integrated contractions of the stomach, pylorus, and duodenum produce a regulated delivery of contents into the small intestine through the process of gastric emptying.

ANATOMICAL CONSIDERATIONS

The gastric component of the emptying process is the result of the activity of smooth muscle cells that are arranged in three layers: an outer longitudinal layer, a middle circular layer, and an inner oblique layer. The longitudinal layer is absent on the anterior and posterior surfaces of the stomach. The circular layer is the most prominent and is present in all areas of the stomach except the paraesophageal region. The oblique layer is the least complete, being formed from two bands of muscle lying on the anterior and posterior surfaces. These two bands meet orally at the gastroesophageal sphincter and fan out to fuse with the circular muscle layer in the caudad part of the stomach. Both the circular and the longitudinal muscle layers increase in thickness toward the duodenum.

The stomach is innervated richly with both intrinsic and extrinsic nerves. The intrinsic nerves lie in various plexuses, the most prominent being the myenteric plexus that lies in a three-dimensional matrix between the longitudinal and circular muscle layers and throughout the circular muscle layer. The myenteric plexus receives nerve endings from other intrinsic plexuses as well as extrinsic nerves. Axons from neurons within the myenteric plexus synapse with the muscle fibers and with glandular cells of the stomach. Extrinsically the stomach is innervated by branches of the vagus nerves and by fibers originating in the celiac plexus of the sympathetic nervous system.

The pylorus, or gastroduodenal junction, is characterized by a thickening of the circular muscle layer of the distal antrum. Separating this bundle of muscle from the duodenum is a connective tissue septum; however, some of the longitudinal muscle fibers pass from the antrum to connect with muscle cells of the duodenum. The pylorus is richly innervated with both extrinsic and intrinsic nerves. In particular, nerve endings within the thickened circular muscle layer are abundant. Many of these contain neuropeptides, especially enkephalin.

The anatomy of the proximal duodenum is similar to that of the rest of the intestine (as described in Chapter 5). One significant difference is the larger number of intrinsic nerves present in this area, as compared to the rest of the small bowel. These may be involved in the regulation of gastric emptying described in the following sections.

CONTRACTIONS OF THE ORAD AREA OF THE STOMACH

This area of the stomach exhibits little contractile activity during the digestive state. A pressure-sensing device placed in the orad stomach detects a resting pressure essentially equal to intraabdominal pressure. Superimposed on this resting pressure are various tonic pressure changes. The predominant changes are low in amplitude and have a duration of 1 minute or more. Another indication of this minimal activity is that little mixing of ingested contents occurs in the orad stomach. The food tends to remain in relatively undisturbed layers for an hour or more after eating. The predominant motor activity in this portion of the stomach, as has been described in the previous chapter, is concerned with the accommodation of ingested material.

As the stomach empties the orad region contracts. Whether the musculature contracts tonically simply to accommodate the remaining gastric contents, or if it contracts to propel material into the caudad stomach is not known. Both gastrin and cholecystokinin decrease contractions and increase the distensibility of the orad region of the stomach. At present, however, only the effect of CCK appears to be physiological.

CONTRACTIONS OF THE CAUDAD REGION OF THE STOMACH

Compared to the orad stomach, the caudad region exhibits marked activity. After eating, contractions of varying amplitudes occur almost continuously. Contractions normally begin in the midstomach and move toward the gastroduodenal junction (Fig. 4-1). As they approach the junction they increase in both force and velocity. Thus the primary contractile event in the caudad stomach is a peristaltic contraction. Between contractions, pressures in the caudad region are near intraabdominal levels. When contractions begin they are seen as rhythmic increases and decreases in pressure. In humans the duration of these contractions ranges between 2 and 20 seconds, and the maximum frequency is 3 to 5 contractions per minute.

Contractions of the caudad region of the stomach serve to both mix and propel gastric contents. As the contraction begins in the midportion of the stomach, gastric contents are propelled in front of the contraction toward the gastroduodenal junction (Fig. 4-2, *A*). As the contraction approaches the junction, some of the contents are evacuated into the duodenum (Fig. 4-2, *B*). The peristaltic wave, however, increases in velocity at a rate faster than the movement of the gastric contents. Once the contractile wave overtakes the contents, most of the contents are propelled back into the main body of the stomach (Fig. 4-2, *C*). This propulsion back into the stomach has been termed "retropulsion." Retropulsion causes a thorough mixing of the gastric contents and mechanically reduces the size of solid particles. Thus the peristaltic contractions of the caudad stomach both mix and empty gastric contents.

Contractions of the caudad area of the stom-

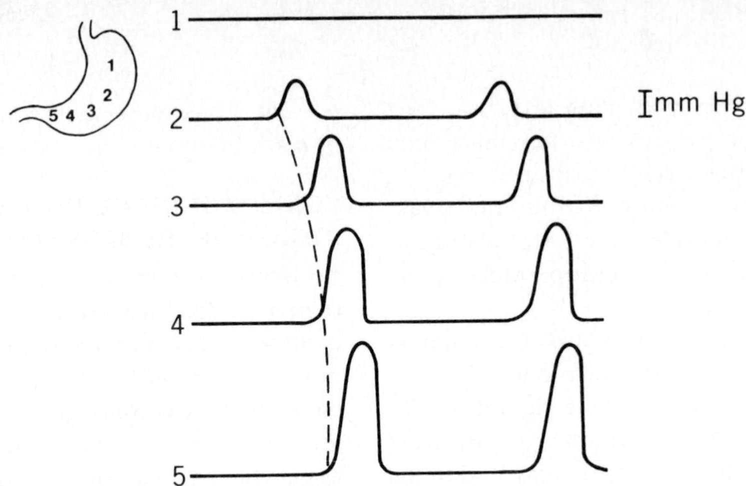

Fig. 4-1. Intraluminal pressures recorded from five areas of the stomach. A sensor in the orad region records little phasic activity. Sensors in the caudad region detect peristaltic contractions, which begin in the midportion of the stomach and progress toward the gastroduodenal junction. The contractions increase in force and velocity as they near the junction and repeat at multiple intervals of from 12 to 20 seconds. The presence and force of contractions depend on the digestive state of the individual.

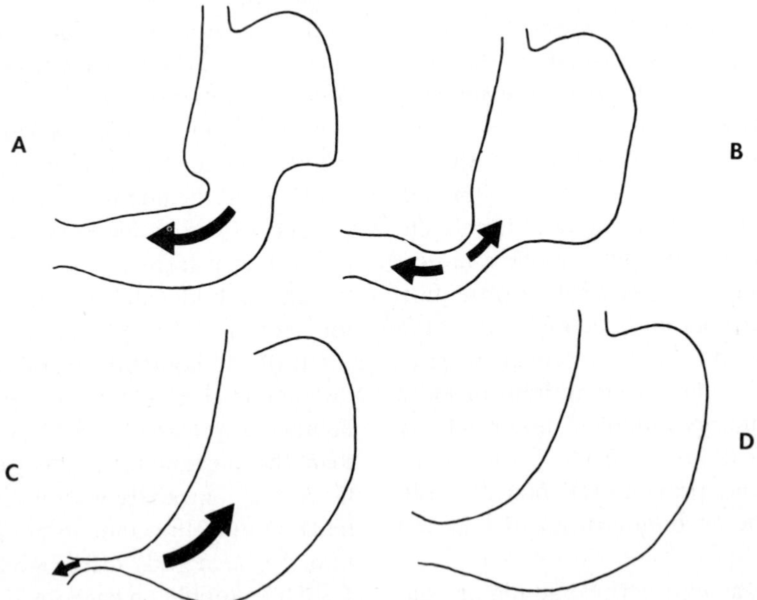

Fig. 4-2. Effects that gastric peristaltic contractions have on intraluminal contents. **A**, The contraction begins in the midregion of the stomach and pushes contents toward the duodenum. **B**, As the contraction increases in force and velocity, some of the contents are passed over and forced back into the body of the stomach. **C**, Contraction force and velocity are great enough to cause rapid and almost complete closure of the distal antrum. Before and during this contraction some contents are propelled into the duodenum. However, most are propelled back into the body of the stomach. **D**, No gross movement of the gastric contents occurs between contractions.

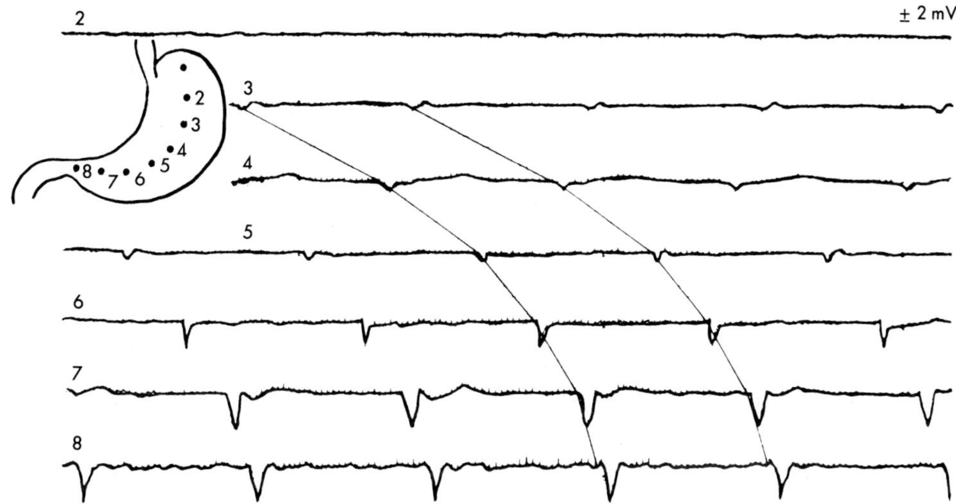

Fig. 4-3. Electrical activity of smooth muscle cells of the stomach. Electrodes placed on the serosal surface record no changes from the orad region. In the midregion, however, slow waves occur continuously at intervals of 12 to 20 seconds. Slow waves give the appearance of moving caudad at increasing velocities. Compare this with Fig. 4-1. *(Adapted from Kelly KA et al: Am J Physiol 217:461-471, 1969.)*

ach are controlled by activities of the smooth muscle cells themselves as well as by nervous and humoral elements. Smooth muscle cells in this area have a membrane potential that fluctuates rhythmically with cyclic depolarizations and repolarizations. These fluctuations are called "slow waves" (also "basic electric rhythm," "pacesetter potentials," and "control activity"). Slow waves have two components: an initial upstroke potential and a secondary plateau potential. In the stomach, slow waves can initiate significant contractions; thus some investigators refer to them as action potentials. However, slow waves are always present, regardless of the presence or absence of contractions. Their frequency is constant; in humans it is between 3 and 5 cycles/min (cpm). If slow waves are recorded from multiple sites between the midstomach and the gastroduodenal junction, they demonstrate the same frequency at all sites (Fig. 4-3). However, slow waves do not occur simultaneously at all points along the stomach. Rather, a phase lag occurs; thus they seem to pass from an area in the midstomach toward the gastroduodenal junction. This phase lag between slow waves at equidistant points lessens as the slow waves approach the gastroduodenal junction. The velocity of the peristaltic wave therefore is controlled by the velocity of spread of the slow wave.

Nervous and humoral factors are not necessary for the presence of slow waves, but they do alter slow wave behavior. Vagotomy disorganizes the slow waves so that the phase lag varies in both duration and direction. The hormone gastrin increases the frequency of gastric slow waves while having little effect on their apparent propagation through the musculature.

Simultaneous recordings of both electrical and mechanical activities have shown that slow waves initiate contractions of the musculature only when the plateau potential exceeds a threshold value (Fig. 4-4). Once the threshold is exceeded, the greater the ampli-

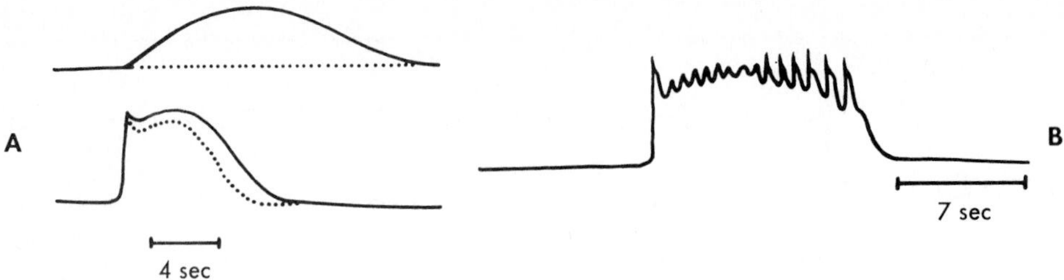

Fig. 4-4. A, Relationship between electrical and mechanical activities of smooth muscle from the caudad region of the stomach. *Bottom tracing* depicts two slow waves (action potentials) superimposed. *Top tracing* depicts mechanical events associated with the potential changes. Note that a contraction is initiated only by the slow wave of larger amplitude and longer duration. **B**, Slow wave potential recorded from distal antrum. Note the oscillations and spike potentials during plateau. *(**A**, Adapted from Szurszewski J: J Physiol 252:335-361, 1975. **B**, Adapted from El-Sharkaway TY et al: J Physiol 279:291-307, 1978.)*

tude of the plateau, the greater will be the force of contraction. The plateau potential may or may not be accompanied by superimposed rapid oscillations called "spike potentials" or "spike bursts." These oscillations also appear to initiate contractions and are seen more frequently in the muscle of the caudad antrum. The threshold for contraction is not reached by every slow wave. Therefore not every slow wave is accompanied by a contraction. If the threshold is reached, it is only during a specific phase of the slow wave cycle. Thus the phasic and peristaltic nature of gastric contractions results from the presence of slow waves.

The amplitude of the plateau potential and, therefore, the number and force of contractions are influenced markedly by nervous and humoral activities. Vagal nerve transection leads to a decrease in contraction, whereas stimulation increases the frequency and force of contractions. Usually sympathetic nerve activity depresses contractions. Some hormones, such as gastrin and motilin, increase contraction, whereas others, such as secretin and GIP, inhibit them. The physiological significance of these actions is not known.

CONTRACTIONS OF THE GASTRODUODENAL JUNCTION

The question of whether a true sphincter exists between the stomach and duodenum is unsettled. There is a definite difference in the contractile activities of the stomach, on one side, and the duodenum, on the other. One contracts at a frequency of 3 to 5 cpm, and the other at 10 to 12 cpm. There is a thickened ring of circular muscle between the two organs that behaves independently. Some investigators have demonstrated a zone of elevated pressure between the stomach and the duodenum in humans (an indication of sphincteric activity); others, however, have not found such an area. Recent studies have shown that even if a zone of elevated pressure is not found, the pylorus can contract independently, thus altering the resistance to flow between the stomach and duodenum (Fig. 4-5). This can have a large effect on gastric emptying.

CONTRACTIONS OF THE PROXIMAL DUODENUM

Duodenal contractions, like those of the caudad region of the stomach, are mostly pha-

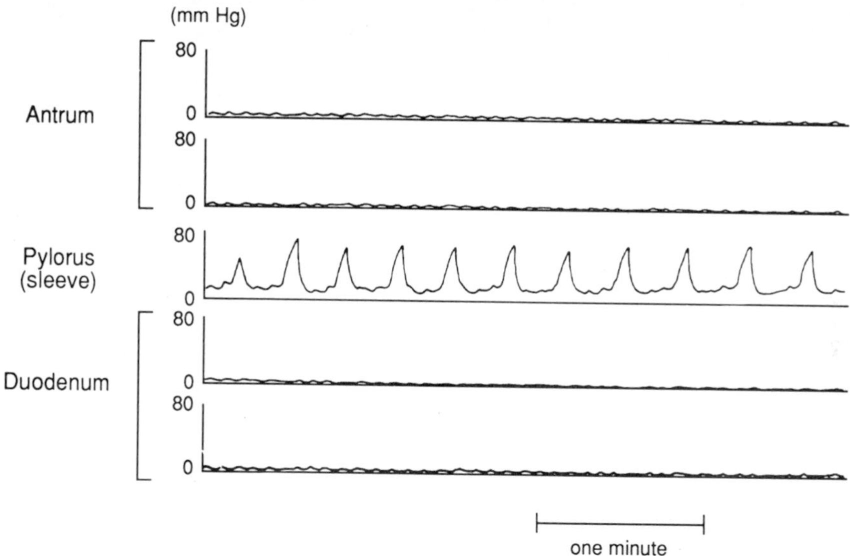

Fig. 4-5. Intraluminal pressures recorded from two areas of the stomach (Antrum), the pylorus, and two areas of the proximal doudenum during the intraduodenal infusion of lipid. Note the regular isolated contractions, and the elevated pressures (*O* indicates atmospheric pressure in each tracing) between contractions in the pylorus. This activity is occurring at a time when there are no contractions present in the stomach and duodenum. *(Adapted from Heddle R et al: Am J Physiol 254:G671-G679, 1988.)*

sic. The maximal frequency of duodenal contractions is much higher, 11 to 12 per minute compared to 3 to 5 per minute in the stomach. However, in the digestive state duodenal contractions seldom occur in a continuous manner. Rather, isolated contractions or small groups of contractions separated by intervals of no contraction are the norm. Also, duodenal contractions are not always peristaltic. As discussed in Chapter 5, most contractions of the small intestine are of the segmenting type. Thus, depending upon their number and pattern, duodenal contractions either impede or facilitate the emptying of contents from the stomach.

REGULATION OF GASTRIC EMPTYING

Immediately after ingestion of a meal the stomach may contain over a liter of material, which then takes several hours to leave the stomach and empty into the small intestine. This process of gastric emptying appears to be regulated in a manner that allows optimum time for digestion and absorption of foodstuffs from the small intestine, and it involves coordinated contractile activity of the stomach, pylorus, and proximal small intestine (Fig. 4-6).

The transfer rate of material from the stomach into the duodenum depends on the physical and chemical composition of the gastric contents (Fig. 4-7). Solids empty only after a lag period during which they are reduced in size by the retropulsive activity of the caudad stomach. Liquids begin to empty almost immediately. The rate of emptying of both solids and liquids depends upon their chemical composition. Material that is high in lipids, H^+, and that deviates markedly in osmotic pressure from that of plasma all empty at a

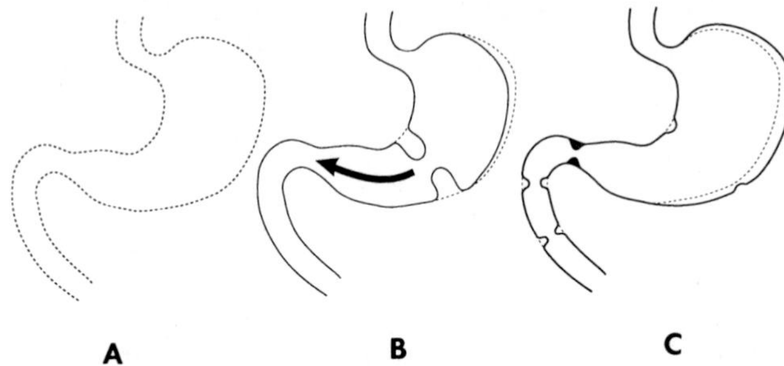

Fig. 4-6. Regulation of gastric emptying. **A,** Hypothetical conditions immediately after the rapid ingestion of a meal and prior to the onset of any contractile activity. This outline is superimposed in **B** and **C** to illustrate changes. **B,** Conditions favoring emptying are increased tone of the orad region of the stomach, forceful peristaltic contractions of the caudad region of the stomach, relaxation of the pylorus, and absence of segmenting contractions of the duodenum. As nutrients emptied from the stomach are further digested and absorbed in the small intestine, they excite receptors located in the intestinal mucosa. Activation of these receptors results in **C**: relaxation of the orad region of the stomach, a decrease in the number and force of contractions of the caudad region of the stomach, contraction of the pylorus, and an increase in segmenting contractions of the duodenum. This results in a slowing of gastric emptying.

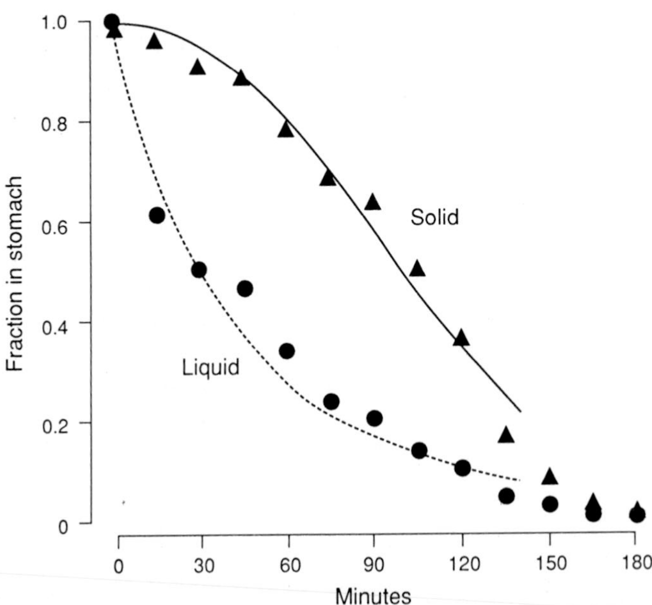

Fig. 4-7. Solid and liquid components of a meal were labeled so that their emptying from the stomach could be followed over time after ingestion of the meal. As indicated by the sharp decrease in the fraction remaining in the stomach, the liquid component began to empty almost immediately, and it emptied more rapidly. On the other hand there was a lag time before the emptying of the label attached to the solid component, and this label emptied more slowly. This slower emptying is attributable to the fact that the solid component had to be reduced to small particles before being emptied into the duodenum. *(Adapted from Camilleri M et al: Am J Physiol 249:G580–585, 1985.)*

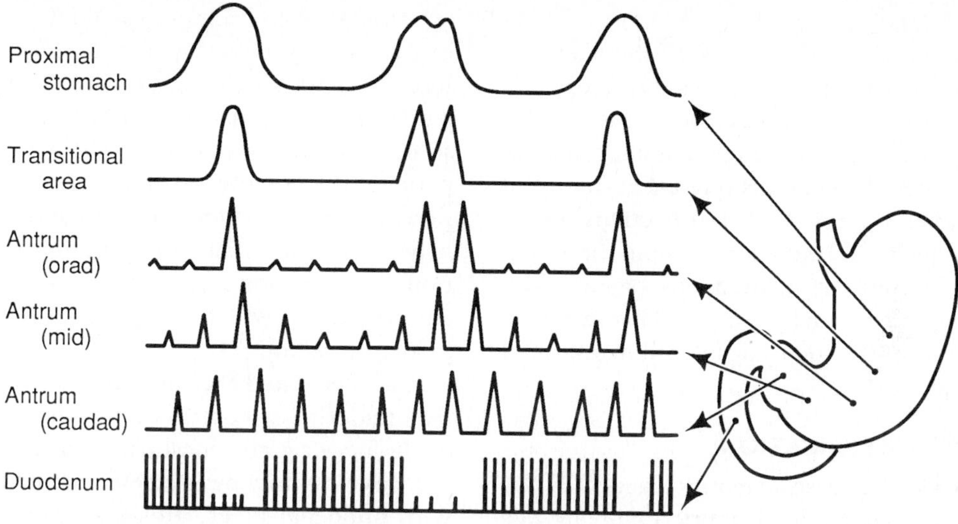

Fig. 4-8. Schematic of intraluminal pressures recorded from the stomach and proximal duodenum during an active phase of a migrating motor complex. Note that phasic contractions begin in the orad region of the stomach and propagate over the caudad region. As contractions of the caudad region approach the gastroduodenal junction the pylorus relaxes (not shown) and doudenal contractions are inhibited momentarily. This allows contents to be swept into the duodenum. Contents are then propelled toward the colon as described in Chapter 5. *(Adapted from Malageda J-R and Azpiroz F: In Schulz SG, Wood JD, and Rauner BB, editors: The gastrointestinal system, Bethesda, 1989, American Psychological Society.)*

slower rate than do near-isotonic saline solutions.

Part of the regulation results from the presence of "receptors" that lie in the upper small bowel. These appear to respond to the physical properties (such as osmotic pressure) and chemical compositions (H^+, lipids) of the chyme. Receptor activation slows emptying through humoral and/or neural pathways. Many of the substances that inhibit gastric emptying also release one or more gastrointestinal hormones; many of the hormones slow gastric emptying when injected into the intestines. It is tempting to speculate that foodstuffs inhibit emptying by releasing hormones, but such a causal relationship is hard to establish. It is just as likely that these receptors regulate emptying by neural mechanisms.

Regulation of gastric emptying is brought about by alterations in motility of the stomach, gastroduodenal junction, and duodenum. Decreases in distensibility of the orad stomach, increases in the force of peristaltic contractions of the caudad stomach, increases in diameter and inhibition of contractions of the pylorus, and inhibition of segmenting contractions of the proximal duodenum all increase the rate of gastric emptying. Upon activation of the duodenal receptors just mentioned, one or more of these contractile activities of the stomach and the duodenum are reversed to slow emptying (see Fig. 4-6).

The pattern of motility of the gastroduodenal area changes after the nutrient components of the meal have been digested and absorbed. Any large particles of undigested residue that remain in the stomach are emptied by a burst of peristaltic contractions as part of the migrating motility complex (Fig. 4-8). During this burst, powerful contractions begin in the previously inactive orad region and sweep the entire length of the stomach. The pylorus dilates during each sweep, and the duodenum relaxes so that resistance to emptying is minimal. Then duodenal contractions sweep the contents onward as discussed in Chapter 5. After this burst of activity the region remains relaxed for an hour or more. Then intermittent contractions begin again, only to end in another burst. This cycle repeats every 90 minutes or so until ingestion of the next meal.

CLINICAL APPLICATIONS

Disorders of gastric motility generally are manifested by a rate of gastric emptying that is either too slow or too fast. This may reflect an abnormality in one or all of the major motor functions of the stomach. When the stomach fails to empty properly it produces complaints of nausea, loss of appetite, and early satiety; often gastric contents may be vomited. The most common form of impaired emptying results from obstruction at the gastric outlet. Examples are gastric cancer and peptic ulcer disease. In the latter, inflammation and scarring associated with the ulcer actually may occlude the gastric lumen at the pylorus. Impaired emptying also can be caused by the absence or disorganization of motor events in the caudad stomach. These phenomena occur in a variety of metabolic disorders such as diabetes mellitus and potassium depletion.

Vagus nerve section (vagotomy) invariably delays gastric emptying of solids. Consequently vagotomy (to decrease acid secretion in peptic ulcer disease) is coupled with surgical alteration of the pylorus (pyloroplasty) or creation of a new gastric outlet (gastroenterostomy) in an attempt to avoid this complication. After such an operation, emptying of liquids generally is accelerated; even with alteration of the gastric outlet, emptying of solids still may be slowed. The majority of patients undergoing this type of surgery experience no other symptoms. However, others may experience diarrhea, sweating, palpitations, cramps, and a variety of other unpleasant symptoms, which result from changes in gastric emptying.

It is speculated that motility abnormalities may underlie or contribute to other diseases of the upper gastrointestinal tract. For example, gastric emptying is accelerated in patients with duodenal ulcer. This may enhance the delivery of gastric acid to the duodenum, perhaps overcoming the ability of the duodenal mucosa to defend itself against injury. Alternatively, in patients with gastric ulcer, gastric emptying appears to be slowed. This may be a situation in which the stomach is more susceptible to injury.

CLINICAL TESTS

For a variety of reasons, motor events in the stomach do not lend themselves to clinical assessment with techniques such as those used in the esophagus. Therefore evaluation of gastric motility often is limited to qualitative observations of gastric emptying provided by x-ray and fluoroscopic evaluation of a barium-filled stomach. Occasionally aspiration of the stomach at a specific interval after installation of an isotonic saline solution will give information regarding gastric emptying. However, quantitative measurements of motility and emptying currently are confined to the research laboratory.

SUGGESTED REFERENCES

Ehrlein HJ and Akkermans LMA: Gastric emptying. In Akkermans LMA, Johnson AG, and Read NW, editors: Gastric and gastroduodenal motility, New York, 1984, Praeger.

Hunt JN and Knox MT: Regulation of gastric emptying. In Code CF, editor: Handbook of physiology, vol 4, Baltimore, 1968, Williams & Wilkins.

Kelly KA: Motility of the stomach and gastroduodenal junction. In Johnson LR, editor: Physiology of the gastrointestinal tract, ed 2, New York, 1981, Raven Press.

Malagelada J-R and Azpiroz F: Determinants of gastric emptying and transit in the small intestine. In Schultz SG, Wood JD, and Rauner BB, editors: Handbook of physiology: the gastrointestinal system, Bethesda, 1989, American Physiological Society.

Meyer JH: Motility of the stomach and gastroduodenal junction. In Johnson LR, editor: Physiology of the gastrointestinal tract, ed 2, New York, 1987, Raven Press.

5 Motility of the Small Intestine

Norman W. Weisbrodt

Motility of the small intestine is organized to optimize the processes of digestion and absorption of nutrients and the aboral propulsion of undigested material. Thus contractions perform at least three functions: (1) mixing of ingested foodstuffs with digestive secretions and enzymes; (2) circulation of all intestinal contents to facilitate contact with the intestinal mucosa; and (3) net propulsion of the intestinal contents in an aboral direction.

ANATOMICAL CONSIDERATIONS

Contractions of the small intestine are caused by activities of two layers of smooth muscle cells: an outer layer with the long axis of the cells arranged longitudinally and an inner layer with the long axis of the cells arranged circularly. In general the circular muscle layer is thicker, and both layers are more abundant in the proximal intestine, decreasing in thickness distally to the level of the ileocecal junction.

The small intestine is richly innervated by elements of the autonomic nervous system. Within the wall of the intestine itself lie neurons, nerve endings, and receptors of the enteric nervous system. These neural elements tend to be concentrated in several plexuses (see Fig. 2-2). The most prominent, the myenteric or Auerbach plexus, lies between the circular and longitudinal smooth muscle cells. Plexal neurons receive input from other neurons within the plexus, from receptors located in the mucosa and muscle walls, and from the central nervous system by way of the parasympathetic and sympathetic nerve trunks. Many neurotransmitters are present in the enteric nervous system, including acetylcholine, norepinephrine, VIP, enkephalin, and other peptides.

Extrinsic innervation is supplied by the vagus nerve and by nerve fibers from the celiac and superior mesenteric ganglia (see Fig. 2-1). Many of the fibers within the vagus are preganglionic, whereas many from the abdominal ganglia are postganglionic. Some of the fibers within the vagus are cholinergic, whereas some from the abdominal plexuses

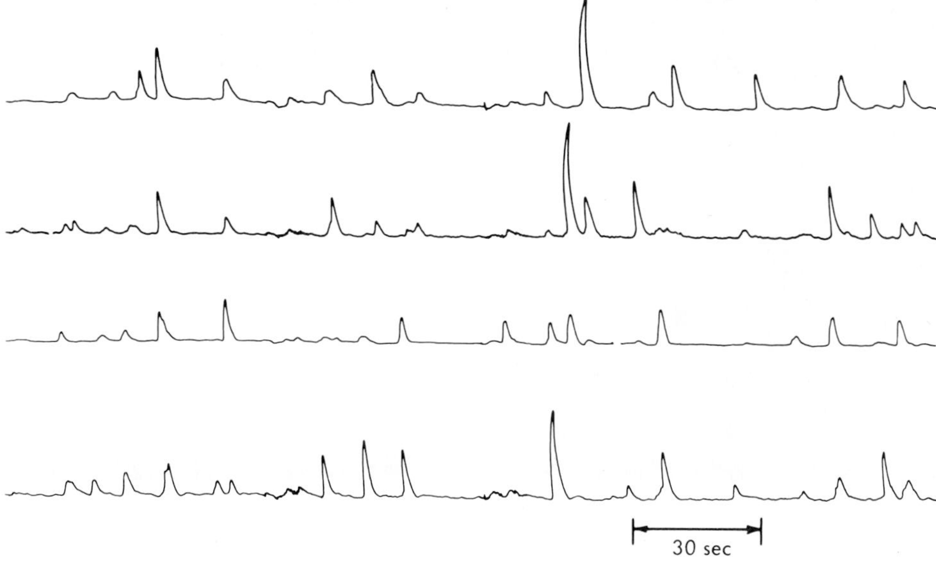

Fig. 5-1. Intraluminal pressure changes recorded from the duodenum of a conscious man. Sensors placed 1 cm apart record changes in pressure that are phasic, lasting 4 to 5 seconds. Note that a rather large contraction can take place at one site while nothing is recorded 1 cm away on either side.

are adrenergic. There is physiological as well as anatomical evidence of other neurotransmitters, which await identification.

TYPES OF CONTRACTIONS

Between contractions, pressures within the lumen of the small intestine approximately equal intraabdominal pressure. When the musculature contracts the lumen is occluded partially or totally, and pressure increases. Most contractions are local events and involve only 1 to 4 cm of bowel at a time. The contractions usually produce intraluminal pressure waves that appear as nearly symmetrical peaks of uniform shape with a mean duration of 5 seconds (Fig. 5-1). In the human upper small bowel they occur at any one site, at multiple intervals of 5 seconds (Fig. 5-2).

Occasionally other types of pressure waves can be recorded. One such type consists of an elevated baseline pressure that lasts from 10 seconds to 8 minutes. This wave seldom occurs alone, usually being accompanied by superimposed phasic changes in pressure.

The effect that any contraction has on intestinal contents depends upon the state of the musculature above and below the point of the contraction. If a contraction is not coordinated with activity above and below, intestinal contents are displaced both proximally and distally during the contraction and may flow back during the period of relaxation. This would serve to mix and locally circulate the contents (Fig. 5-3). Such contractions appear to divide the bowel into segments, which accounts for the name "segmentation" given to this process. If, however, the contractions at adjacent sites occur in a proximal-to-distal sequence, aboral propulsion will result.

The small intestine also is capable of eliciting a highly coordinated contractile response that is propulsive in function. When an area of bowel is stimulated (for example, by placement of a bolus of material in the lumen) the

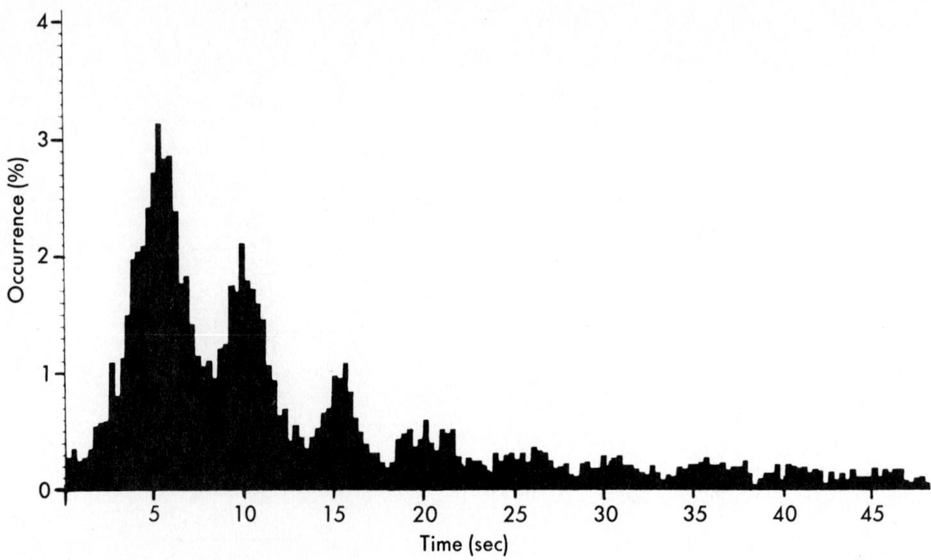

Fig. 5-2. Frequency distribution of 7572 contractions recorded at one site in the human small intestine. Note that the contractions are most frequent at multiples of 5 seconds, which is the approximate interval between slow waves in this region. *(From Christensen J et al: Am J Physiol 221:1818-1823, 1971.)*

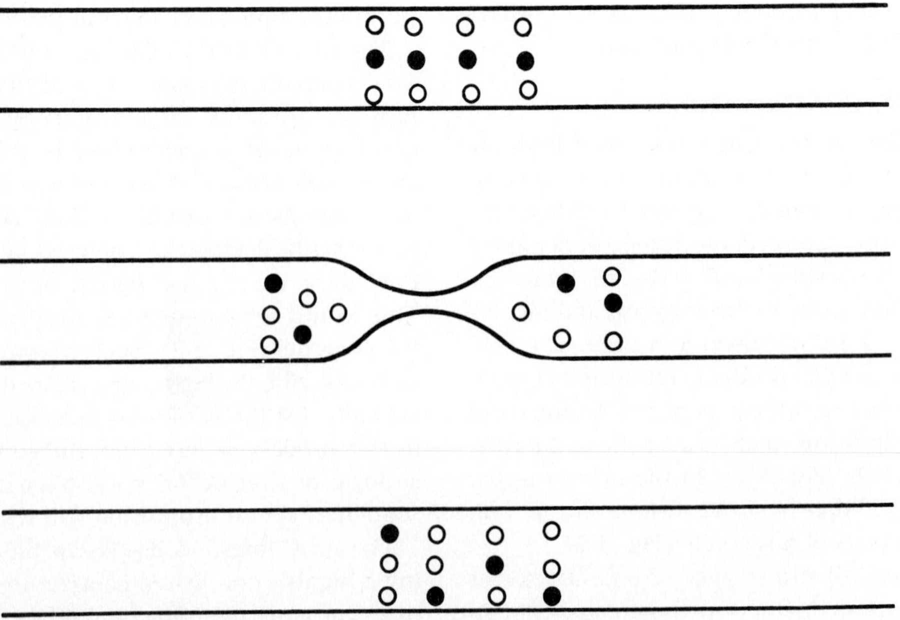

Fig. 5-3. Contractions that are neither preceded nor followed by other contractions serve to mix and locally circulate the intestinal contents.

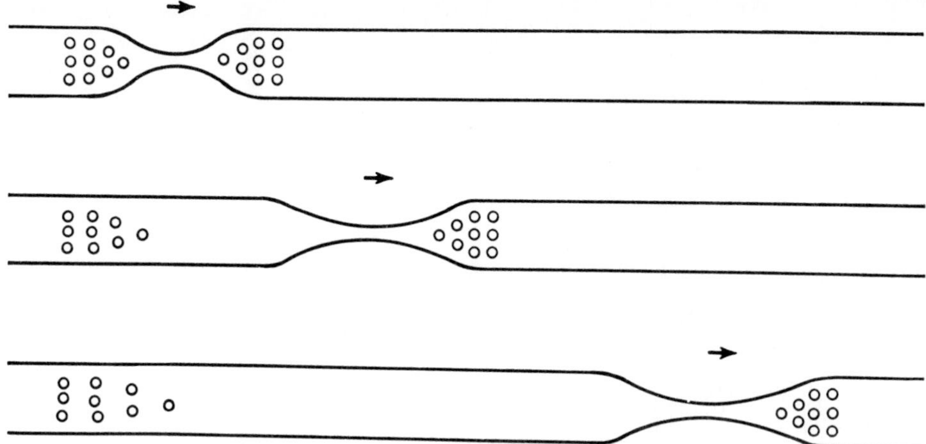

Fig. 5-4. Contractions that have an orad-to-aboral sequence *(left-to-right)* serve to propel contents in a net aboral direction.

bowel responds with contraction orad and relaxation aborad to the point of stimulation. These events tend to move the material in an aboral direction (Fig. 5-4), and if they occur sequentially they can propel a bolus the entire length of the gut in a short time. This peristaltic response, first described by Bayliss and Starling, is known as the "law of the intestines." Often it is invoked to explain how material normally is propelled through the small bowel. Recently, however, its importance in healthy individuals has been downgraded. Peristalsis involving long segments of intestine is seldom seen in normal individuals, although short (1- to 4-cm) peristaltic contractions have been described.

PATTERNS OF CONTRACTIONS

Not only are there differences in individual contractions of the intestine, there are also different patterns of contractions. In the fasting human, contractions do not occur evenly over time. Rather, at any one locus there are cycles of no or few contractions followed by intense sequential contractions. Such cycles repeat about every 1.5 hours (Fig. 5-5). The cycle length is the same at all loci; however, the 5- to 10-minute periods of intense contractions do not occur simultaneously at all points along the intestine. Instead, these groups occur on sequential segments and thus appear to migrate aborally. It takes approximately 1.5 hours to sweep from the duodenum through the ileum. The characteristics of this pattern have earned it the title of "migrating motor complex" (MMC). As discussed in Chapter 4, this complex begins in the stomach and sweeps undigested contents from the stomach, through the small intestine, and into the colon.

In a nonfasting individual, contractions are spread more uniformly over time. They are present 14% to 34% of the recorded time, with the most common pattern being one to three sequential contractions separated by periods of 5, 10, 15, or 20 seconds.

Contractions of the intestine are controlled by activities of the smooth muscle cells themselves as well as by nerves and humoral substances. As in the stomach, smooth muscle cells in the small intestine have a membrane potential that fluctuates rhythmically with cy-

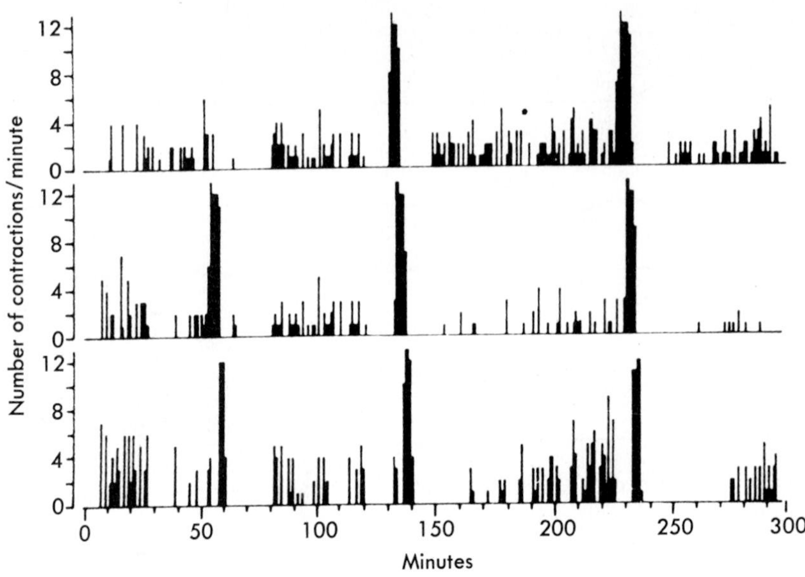

Fig. 5-5. Contractions at three loci in the small bowel. The number of contractions in each minute of the recording were counted and plotted against the time of recording. The resulting histogram indicates cycles of activity at each locus. Also, the periods of intense contractions appear to migrate aborally along the bowel. Such a pattern is called the "migrating motor complex." *(From Vantrappen G et al: J Clin Invest 59:1158-1166, 1977.)*

clic depolarizations and repolarizations of 5 to 15 mV (Fig. 5-6). This slow wave activity (or basic electrical rhythm) is always present whether contractions are occurring or not. At any one site in the intestine, slow wave frequency is constant. Frequency, however, is not the same at all levels of the bowel. There is a decrease in frequency toward the ileocecal junction. In humans the frequency decreases from a mean of 11 or 12 cpm in the duodenum to 8 or 9 cpm in the terminal ileum. The decrease is not linear because frequency is constant throughout the duodenum and for about 10 cm into the jejunum. Beyond that point it declines more or less linearly.

Although slow wave frequency is identical over the proximal small intestine, slow waves do not occur simultaneously at all points. Multiple electrodes detect a proximal-to-distal phase lag that simulates a propagated signal (Fig. 5-6).

In the small intestine, slow waves themselves do not initiate significant contractions. Contractions are initiated by a second electrical event, often referred to as "spike potential activity." This consists of rapid depolarizations of the membrane that appear to be superimposed on the depolarization phase of the slow wave. At any one site spike potentials do not occur with every slow wave. When they do occur, they tend to be localized. An electrode placed 1 to 2 cm on either side of an active area may detect slow waves only. Slow waves, spike potentials, and contractions are interrelated. Spike potentials always precede a contraction, and they occur during specific periods of the slow wave cycle; therefore the slow wave determines the timing of contractions, and contractions occur at multiples of the slow wave interval. Thus it is no coincidence that in the human proximal bowel

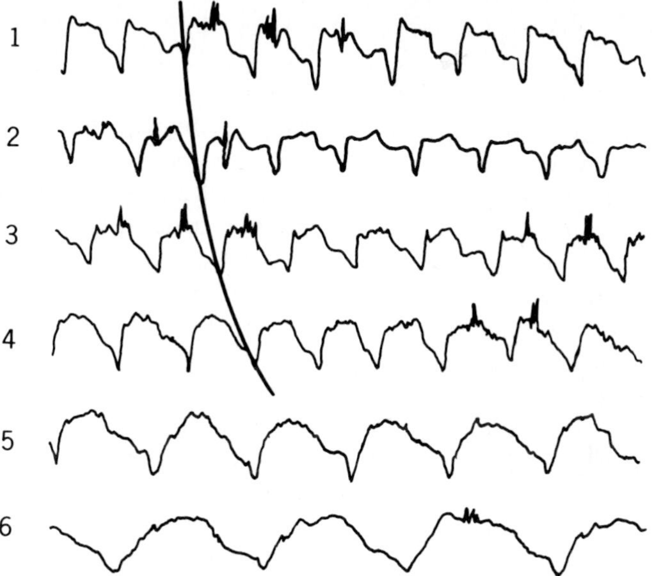

Fig. 5-6. Slow waves and spike potentials from multiple sites in the small intestine. Tracings *1* to *6* illustrate activity from progressively distal areas. *Solid line* connecting the slow waves in tracings *1* to *4* denotes the apparent propagation in the region of a slow-wave frequency plateau. Tracings *5* and *6* show decreases in slow-wave frequency at more distal areas. The rapid transients that occur on the peaks of some of the slow waves represent spike potentials.

slow waves occur every 5 seconds and contractions occur at intervals lasting for multiples of 5 seconds. Also, because a gradient exists in the slow wave frequency along the small bowel, there is a gradient in the maximal frequency of contractions.

Besides determining the temporal relationships of contractions at one site in the bowel, slow waves also influence the spatial relationships of contractions at adjacent sites. The phase lag in occurrence of slow waves at adjacent sites imposes a phase lag in the occurrence of contractions at adjacent sites. Thus it is not surprising to learn that a peristaltic contraction moves at the same velocity as the apparent velocity of the slow wave.

Although slow waves determine the timing of contractions they do not determine whether spike potentials and contractions will occur. Occurrence of contractions depends on nervous activity and circulating or local chemical agents. There are a number of reflexes that depend upon the intrinsic neurons, the extrinsic neurons, or both. The peristaltic reflex (law of the intestines) described previously depends on an intact enteric nervous system. Application of neural blocking agents will abolish or greatly reduce this reflex. Another reflex, the intestino-intestinal reflex, depends upon extrinsic neural connections. If an area of the bowel is distended grossly, contractile activity in the rest of the bowel is inhibited. Sectioning of the extrinsic nerves abolishes this reflex. Additionally, it is well known that changes in the emotional state of an individual can induce alterations in small-bowel motility. Thus the small bowel is under the influence of higher centers of the nervous system.

In addition to neural control, many circulating and endogenously released chemicals alter intestinal motility. Epinephrine released from the adrenal glands tends to inhibit contractions. Serotonin, which is contained in large quantities within the small intestine, stimulates contractions, as do certain of the prostaglandins. Several hormones also alter intestinal motility. Gastrin, CCK, motilin, and insulin tend to stimulate contractions, whereas secretin and glucagon tend to inhibit them. The exact role of these chemical agents in the regulation of motility has yet to be clarified.

The presence of a distinct pattern of contractions during fasting (the MMC) indicates complex controlling mechanisms. Segments of intestine that have been denervated extrinsically still exhibit MMCs. Thus the enteric nervous system may regulate its periodicity and apparent migration. However, the hormone motilin is released endogenously with the same periodicity as the phase of contractions of the MMC, and exogenously administered motilin will initiate a premature MMC. Thus MMCs may be modulated by hormones and the activity of extrinsic nerves. Feeding abolishes MMCs and institutes a pattern of more or less continuous contractions of varying amplitude. The change in pattern with feeding probably is brought about by both humoral and neural mechanisms.

CLINCAL APPLICATION

Primary disorders of small intestinal motility probably are rare. The small intestine may be involved in certain general disorders of the smooth muscle of the gastrointestinal and urinary tracts. The cause of these disorders is unknown, but in some patients there may be a genetic basis. When the disorder is clinically apparent the patient appears to have episodes of intestinal obstruction; however, the problem seems to involve failure of propulsive motility rather than obstruction. Thus the name "idiopathic pseudo-obstruction" has been coined. In some patients with this syndrome the smooth muscle cells are involved. In others, histological studies show changes in enteric nerves rather than in smooth muscle.

Altered small-intestinal motility resulting in delayed transit frequently accompanies a variety of diseases and clinical situations. Perhaps the most common is the transient ileus or apparent paralysis of the small intestine sometimes seen after abdominal surgery. However, intraabdominal inflammation (pancreatitis, appendicitis, abscess, etc.) may produce a similar picture. Systemic diseases such as diabetes mellitus and amyloidosis, metabolic alterations such as potassium depletion, and administration of drugs, particularly anticholinergics, all may have an adverse effect on intestinal transit. Mixing is likely to be impaired as well, although this is less clinically apparent.

Alternatively, rapid intestinal transit is seen in certain malabsorptive states induced by infectious agents, allergic reaction, and various pharmacological agents. In these conditions both motility and absorption are affected. In most disease states it is not clear whether changes in motility are primary (caused by the disease) or secondary (caused by the presence of unabsorbed or secreted material). Also the contractile events and patterns of motility that underlie these conditions remain largely unknown.

CLINICAL TESTS

Because of the inaccessibility of the small intestine, direct measurement of contractions or electrical activity is extremely difficult and, as yet, not employed routinely. Often auscultation to detect "sounds" is used to assess bowel activity. In addition, observing the movement of barium can yield some information on transit time through the small bowel. Unfortunately, however, the wide range of normal values for intestinal transit makes it difficult to utilize transit time as a diagnostic tool unless transit is altered markedly.

SUGGESTED REFERENCES

Vantrappen G, Janssens J, and Peeters TL: The migrating motor complex, Med Clin 65:1313-1321, 1981.

Weisbrodt NW: Motility of the small intestine. In Johnson LR, editor: Physiology of the gastrointestinal tract, ed 2, New York, 1987, Raven Press.

Wingate DL: Backward and forward with the migrating complex, Dig Dis Sci 26:641-666, 1981.

6 Motility of the Large Intestine

Norman W. Weisbrodt

Contractions of the large intestine are organized to allow for optimum absorption of water and electrolytes, net aboral movement of contents, and the storage and orderly evacuation of feces.

ANATOMICAL CONSIDERATIONS

Anatomically the human large intestine is divided into the cecum; the ascending, transverse, descending, and sigmoid colons; the rectum; and the anal canal. The muscular layers of the large intestine are composed of both longitudinally and circularly arranged fibers. Longitudinal fibers are concentrated into three flat bands called the taeniae coli. These run from the cecum to the rectum, where the fibers fan out to form a more continuous longitudinal coat. The circular layer of muscle fibers is continuous from the cecum to the anal canal, where it increase in thickness to form the internal anal sphincter. Overlapping and slightly distal to the internal anal sphincter are layers of striated muscle. These striated muscle bundles make up the external anal sphincter.

In humans the external features of the large intestine differ from those of the small intestine. In addition to the presence of taeniae coli, the colon appears to be divided into segments called "haustra" or "haustrations" (Fig. 6-1). Haustra are probably the result of structural and functional properties of the colon. Points of concentration of muscular tissue and mucosal foldings can be found in colons examined postmortem. Also haustra are more prominent in areas of the colon that possess taeniae coli. Haustra are not fixed, however. Segmental colonic contractions appear, disappear, and re-form at another locus. Thus haustral formation also has a dynamic component because of the contractile activity of colonic musculature.

The large intestine, like other areas of the bowel, is innervated by the autonomic nervous system. The enteric system consists partly of many nerve cell bodies and endings that lie between the circular and longitudinal muscle coats. In areas of the large intestine with taeniae this myenteric plexus is concentrated beneath them. Cells of the myenteric

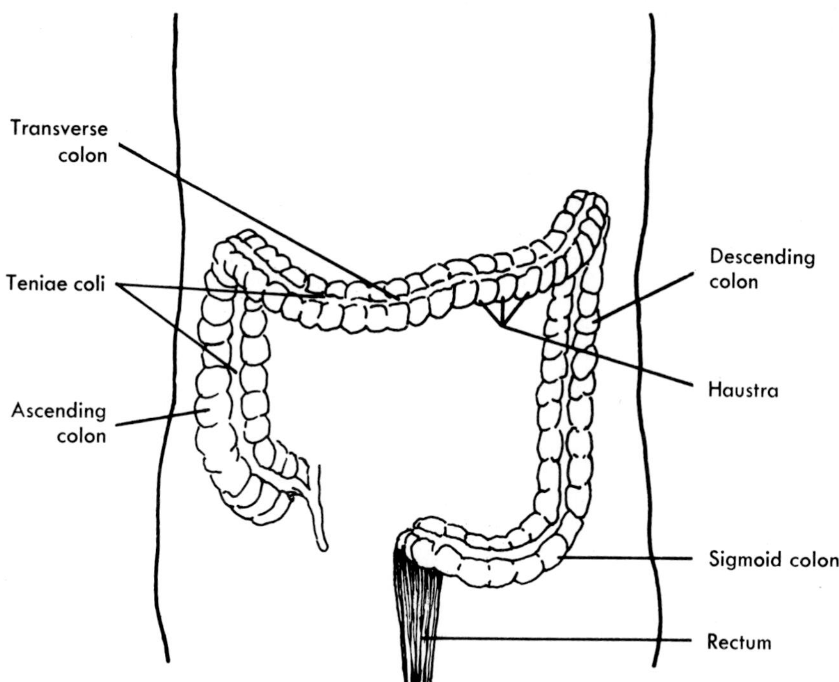

Fig. 6-1. Anatomy of the colon. Note that it is short and large in diameter when compared to the small intestine. The longitudinal smooth muscle is concentrated into three bands *(taeniae coli)* in all regions except the rectum. Note also that all regions except the rectum possess *haustra*. The exact cause of haustration is not known. They are formed partly by contractions of the circular muscle; however, because they are still present after death, some investigators believe they have a permanent structural basis.

plexus receive input from a variety of receptors within the intestine as well as input by way of the extrinsic nerves. Axons from these cells innervate the muscle layers. Extrinsic innervation of the large intestine comes from both parasympathetic and sympathetic branches of the autonomic nervous system. There are two pathways of parasympathetic innervation: the cecum and the ascending and transverse portions of the colon are innervated by the vagus nerve; the descending and sigmoid areas of the colon and the rectum are innervated by pelvic nerves from the sacral region of the spinal cord. The vagus and pelvic nerves consist primarily of preganglionic efferent fibers and many afferent fibers. The efferent fibers supposedly synapse with the nerve cell bodies of the myenteric and other intrinsic plexuses. The proximal regions of the large intestine are sympathetically innervated by fibers that come from the superior mesenteric ganglion. More distal regions receive input from the inferior mesenteric ganglion. The distal rectum and anal canal are innervated by sympathetic fibers from the hypogastric plexus. Most of the sympathetic fibers are postganglionic efferent and afferent fibers. The external anal sphincter, a striated muscle, is innervated by the somatic pudendal nerves.

Acetylcholine and norepinephrine serve as mediators at many of the presynaptic and postsynaptic junctions within the autonomic innervation of the large intestine. There is evidence, however, for several peptide neurocrines and other as yet unidentified neurotransmitters. Transmission between the pudendal nerves and the external anal sphincter is mediated by acetylcholine.

CONTRACTIONS OF THE CECUM AND ASCENDING COLON

Flow of contents from the small intestine into the large intestine is intermittent and regulated partly by a sphincteric mechanism at the ileocecal junction. A sensor placed in the junction records pressures that are several millimeters of mercury greater than those in the ileum or colon. The pressure, however, is not constant, for the sphincter relaxes periodically; during this time ileal contractions propel contents into the large intestine (Fig. 6-2, *A*). Once material reaches the proximal large intestine it is acted on by a wide variety of contractions. The majority of these are segmental in nature, with durations of 12 to 60 seconds. The pressures generated by these contractions vary in amplitude between about 10 and 50 mm Hg. It is believed that these contractions are partly responsible for the haustrations seen in the colon. At adjacent sites contractions usually occur independently. Thus they slowly move the contents back and forth, mixing and exposing them to the mucosa for absorption of water and electrolytes. In addition to pressure changes caused by segmental contractions, a large variety of other pressure waves has been recorded. Attempts to classify these have been made, but the degree of overlap of pressure profiles makes classification difficult.

Occasionally segmental contractions are organized in an orad-to-aborad direction; thus propulsion over short distances takes place. Most propulsion, however, occurs during a characteristic sequence termed "mass movement." Segmental activity suddenly ceases, and along with its disappearance there is a loss of haustrations. The colon then undergoes a contraction that sweeps intraluminal contents in an aborad direction (Fig. 6-3, *A* to *C*). Following the mass movement, haustrations and phasic contractions return (Fig. 6-3, *D*). Mass movements are infrequent in healthy people and are estimated to occur only one to three times daily. Because they are such infrequent events they have not been studied in any great detail in normal individuals.

CONTRACTIONS OF THE DESCENDING AND SIGMOID COLON

By the time material reaches the descending and sigmoid colon, it has changed from a liquid to a semisolid state. Although there is less absorption of water and electrolytes from these portions of the colon, motility studies have demonstrated that contractions of the segmenting type are more frequent here than in the ascending and transverse colon. These segmenting contractions do not result in propulsion. On the contrary they offer resistance and thus retard the flow of contents from more proximal regions into the rectum. Propulsion through these areas probably occurs also during mass movements. Here, too, there is loss of segmental activity and the haustrations that precede transport (Fig. 6-3, *E* and *F*). Thus material that enters these regions during a mass movement is acted on to further reduce its liquid content and is then propelled into the rectum during a subsequent mass movement.

MOTILITY OF THE RECTUM AND ANAL CANAL

The rectum is usually empty or nearly so. Although little material is present, contractions do occur in this region. In fact the upper regions of the rectum contract segmentally more frequently than does the sigmoid colon.

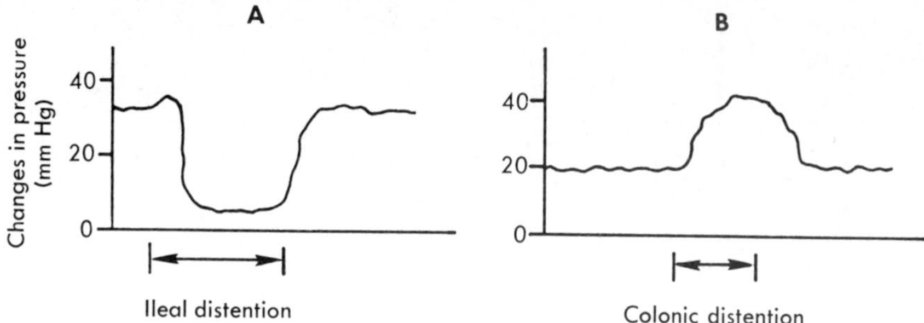

Fig. 6-2. Intraluminal pressures recorded at the level of the ileocecal sphincter. Note that a resting pressure of 20 to 40 mm Hg exists. **A**, Distention of the ileum causes sphincteric relaxation and thus allows flow of contents from the ileum into the colon. **B**, Distention of the colon, on the other hand, causes contraction of the sphincter to prevent passage of contents from the colon to the ileum. *(From Cohen S et al: Gastroenterology 54:72-75, 1968.)*

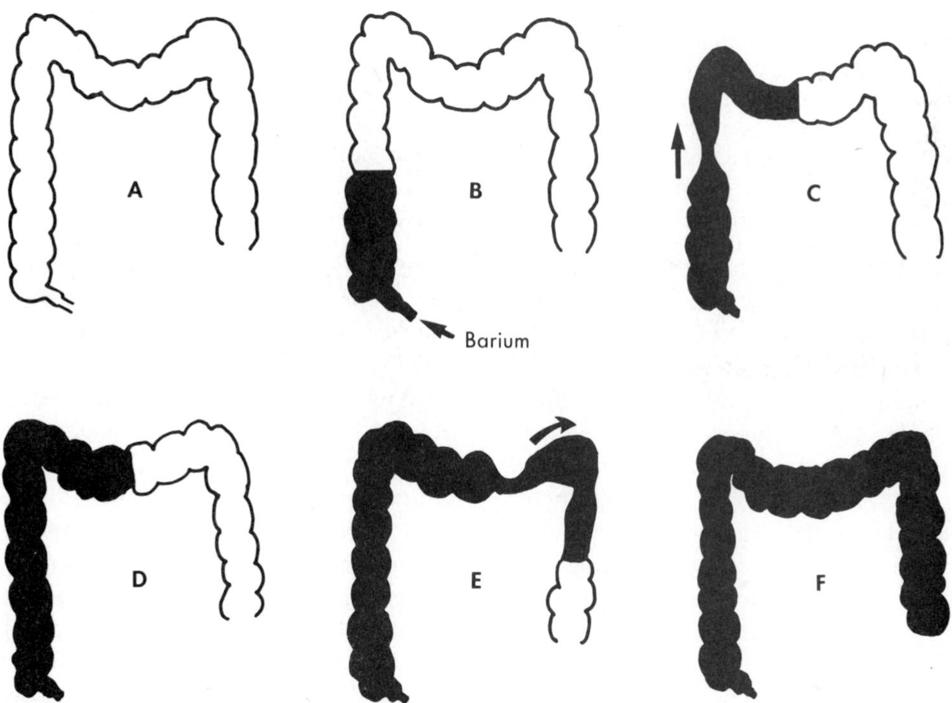

Fig. 6-3. Two mass movements. **A**, Appearance of the colon before the entry of barium sulfate. **B**, As the barium enters from the ileum, it is acted on by haustral contractions. **C**, As more barium enters a portion is swept into and through an area of the colon that has lost its haustral markings. **D**, The barium is acted on by the haustral contractions that have returned. **E**, A second mass movement propels the barium into and through areas of the transverse and descending colon. **F**, Haustrations again return. Most of the movement of feces through the colon is accomplished by this type of contraction.

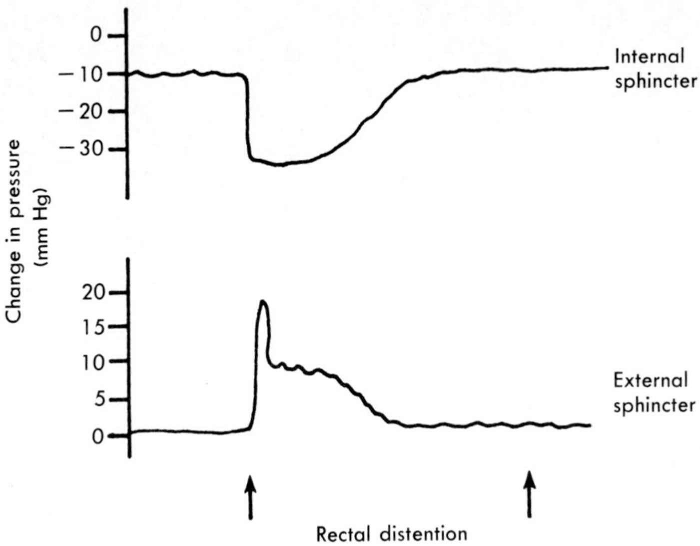

Fig. 6-4. Intraluminal pressure recorded at the level of the internal and external anal sphincters. Although not indicated, a resting pressure of 20 to 30 mm Hg is recorded. Rectal distention causes relaxation of the internal sphincter and contraction of the external sphincter. Note, however, that the changes in sphincteric pressures are transient even though rectal distention is maintained. This is related to the accommodation of the stretch receptors within the wall of the rectum. *(From Schuster MM: Johns Hopkins Med J 116:70-88, 1965.)*

This activity tends to retard the flow of contents into the rectum. When the rectum fills it does so intermittently. During a mass movement or during an aborally directed sequence of segmental contractions of the sigmoid colon, some material passes into the rectum.

Normally the anal canal is closed because of contraction of the internal anal sphincter. When the rectum is distended by fecal material, however, the internal sphincter relaxes as part of the rectosphincteric reflex (Fig. 6-4). Rectal distention also elicits a sensation that signals the urge for defecation. If environmental conditions are not conducive to defecation, voluntary contractions of the external sphincter can overcome the reflex. Relaxation of the internal sphincter is transient because the receptors within the rectal wall accommodate the stimulus of distention. Thus the internal anal sphincter regains its tone, and the sensation subsides until the passage of more contents into the rectum. The rectum can accommodate rather large quantities of material, so it acts as a storage organ.

If the rectosphincteric reflex is elicited at a time when evacuation is convenient, defecation will occur. Defecation is accomplished by a series of voluntary and involuntary acts. When rectal distention is followed by defecation, muscles of the descending and sigmoid colon and the rectum may contract to propel contents toward the anal canal. Then both internal and external sphincters relax to allow passage of the bolus. Normally these events are accompanied by voluntary acts that raise intraabdominal pressure and lower the pelvic floor. Intraabdominal pressure is increased by contractions of the diaphragm and musculature of the abdominal wall. Simultaneously the musculature of the pelvic floor relaxes to allow the increased abdominal pressure to force the floor downward.

CONTROL OF MOTILITY

The factors that control motility of the large intestine are complex and poorly understood. As in the stomach and small intestine, motility in the large intestine is influenced by at least four factors: intrinsic smooth muscle properties, enteric nerves, extrinsic nerves, and circulating or locally released chemicals.

Tone of the ileocecal sphincter is basically myogenic. It is modified, however, by nervous and humoral factors. Distention of the colon causes an increase in sphincteric tension, a reflex probably mediated via the enteric nerves (Fig. 6-2, *B*). Distention of the ileum causes relaxation, also probably mediated via the enteric nerves (Fig. 6-2, *A*). Relaxation of the sphincter and an increase in the contractile activity of the ileum occur with or shortly after eating. This has been termed the gastroileal reflex. One view is that it is mediated by the gastrointestinal hormones, primarily gastrin. Gastrin will cause an increase in the contractile activity of the ileum as well as a relaxation of the ileocecal sphincter. Some investigators, however, feel that this reflex is mediated via the extrinsic autonomic nerves to the intestine.

Smooth muscle cells of the ascending, transverse, descending, and sigmoid colon and of the rectum exhibit fluctuations in their membrane potential. Cyclic depolarizations and repolarizations that possess some of the characteristics of small intestinal slow waves can be recorded. Potential changes that resemble spike potentials also are recorded. These probably initiate contractions, but the exact relationships between changes in potential and contractile activity have not been clarified. In addition, investigators have recorded various oscillations in membrane potential that fit descriptions of neither slow-wave nor spike-potential activities.

Enteric neurons probably are involved in the control of colonic contractions. A peristaltic reflex can be initiated in the colon, and this reflex is mediated by nerve elements within the myenteric plexus. These plexal nerves seem to be predominantly inhibitory, because in their absence the colon is contracted tonically. A number of colonic reflexes have their pathways in the extrinsic nerves. Distention of remote areas of the bowels induces an inhibition of contractions. The pathway for this reflex includes the inferior mesenteric ganglion and also may include the spinal cord. In addition, several investigations have demonstrated that the emotional state of an individual has a marked influence on colonic motility. These influences are mediated by the extrinsic nerves.

Gastrointestinal hormones as well as epinephrine and the prostaglandins affect colonic motility. Gastrin causes an increase in colonic activity and has been implicated in the mass movement that sometimes is seen after eating. Epinephrine causes inhibition of all contractile activity, whereas the prostaglandins (primarily E type) cause a decrease in segmenting contractions and an increase in propulsive activity. The importance of these agents in regulating colonic motility is not known.

The rectosphincteric reflex and the act of defecation are under neural control. Part of the control lies in the enteric nervous system. The reflex, however, is reinforced by activity of neurons within the spinal cord. Destruction of the nerves to the anorectal area can result in fecal retention. The sensation of rectal distention as well as voluntary control of the external anal sphincter are mediated by pathways within the spinal cord to the cerebral cortex. Destruction of these pathways will lead to a loss of voluntary control of defecation.

CLINICAL SIGNIFICANCE

Abnormal transit of material through the colon is common. Delayed transit leads to constipation; in most situations, however, this is dietary in origin. There is a direct correlation between increased dietary fiber, increased colonic intraluminal bulk, and enhanced transit through the colon. How motility of the colon contributes to these changes in transit is not known. A particularly interesting and dramatic clinical disorder in which severe constipation is seen is congenital megacolon (Hirschsprung's disease), characterized by an absence of the enteric nervous system in the distal colon. The internal anal sphincter always is involved, and often the disease extends proximally into the rectum. The involved segment exhibits increased tone, has a very narrow lumen, and is devoid of propulsive activity. As a result the colon proximal to the diseased segment becomes dilated, thus producing a megacolon. This condition is treated through surgical removal of the diseased segment.

In adults the most common gastrointestinal disorder for which medical advice is sought is the irritable bowel syndrome. This disorder gives rise most often to abdominal pain and altered bowel habit (constipation and/or diarrhea). In limited observations, exaggerated segmental contractions in the sigmoid colon have been seen, particularly in response to stimulants such as morphine. During stress, patients with irritable bowel syndrome and constipation exhibit increased segmentation in the sigmoid colon, whereas those with diarrhea exhibit decreased segmentation. The cause of this disorder remains unknown. One theory suggests that altered motility may reflect the conditioning of autonomic responses from repeated exposure to stressful situations. Other investigators have suggested changes in myoelectric activity that might render the colon more susceptible to exogenous influences (stress, drugs, hormones, etc.).

In older age groups, diverticula (outpouchings of mucosa that extend through the muscular wall) frequently develop in the colon. There is evidence to suggest that abnormal colonic motility leads to diverticula formation because of the generation of increased intraluminal pressure. However, a direct correlation between abnormal motility, symptoms, and the presence of diverticula cannot always be demonstrated.

CLINICAL TESTS

Despite the large numbers of patients in whom disordered colonic motility is suspected, techniques for monitoring contractions are not in general clinical use. Most often, radiological procedures are used to provide limited information. However, measurements of intraluminal pressures and myoelectric activity are feasible, especially in the sigmoid colon and rectum, because these areas are readily accessible. To date, such techniques are being used only in investigative studies; their usefulness in diagnosis and the assessment of treatment has yet to be proved.

The behavior of both the internal and the external anal sphincter and the response to rectal distention can be measured by the careful placement of small intraluminal balloons in the anal canal. A third balloon is placed in the rectum and distended to monitor the components of the defecation reflex. This technique has usefulness in patients with suspected neurological disorders that result in impaired defecation.

SUGGESTED REFERENCES

Christensen J: Motility of the colon. In Johnson LR, editor: Physiology of the gastrointestinal tract, ed 2, New York, 1987, Raven Press.

Cohen S, Long WB, and Snape WJ Jr: Gastrointestinal motility. In Guyton AC and Crane RK, editors: Gastrointestinal physiology, vol 3, Baltimore, 1979, University Park Press.

Sanders KM, and Smith TK: Electrophysiology of colonic smooth muscle. In Schultz SG, Wood JD, and Rauner BB, editors: Handbook of physiology: the gastrointestinal system, Bethesda, 1989, American Physiological Society.

7 Salivary Secretion

Leonard R. Johnson

Although the salivary glands are not essential to life, their secretions are important to the hygiene and comfort of the mouth and teeth. The functions of saliva may be divided into those concerned with lubrication, protection, and digestion. An active process produces saliva in large quantities relative to the weights of the salivary glands. Saliva is hyposmotic at all rates of secretion, and unlike the other gastrointestinal secretions, the rate of secretion is almost totally under the control of the nervous system. Another characteristic of this regulation is that both branches of the autonomic nervous system stimulate secretion. The parasympathetic system, however, provides a much greater stimulus than does the sympathetic.

FUNCTIONS OF SALIVA

The lubricating ability of saliva depends primarily on its content of mucus. In the mouth, mixing saliva with food lubricates the ingested material and facilitates the swallowing process. The lubricating effect of saliva is also necessary for speech, as evidenced by the glass of water normally found on the podium of a public speaker.

Saliva exerts its effects through a variety of different mechanisms. It protects the mouth by buffering and diluting noxious substances. Hot solutions of tea, coffee, or soup, for example, are diluted and cooled by saliva. Foul-tasting substances can be washed from the mouth by copious salivation. Similarly the salivary glands are stimulated strongly before vomiting. The corrosive gastric acid and pepsin that are brought up into the esophagus and mouth are thereby neutralized and diluted by saliva. Dry mouth, or xerostomia, is associated with chronic infections of the buccal mucosa and with dental caries. Saliva dissolves and washes out food particles from between the teeth. A number of specialized constituents of saliva have antibacterial actions. These include a lysozyme that attacks bacterial cell walls; lactoferrin, which chelates iron, preventing the multiplication of organisms that require it for growth; and the binding glycoprotein for IgA, which with IgA forms secretory IgA that in turn is immunologically active against viruses and bacteria. Various inorganic compounds are taken up by the salivary glands, concentrated, and secreted in saliva. These include substances such as fluoride and calcium, which subsequently are incorporated into the teeth.

The contributions made by saliva to normal digestion include dissolving and washing away food particles on the taste buds to enable one to taste the next morsel of food eaten. Saliva contains two enzymes, one directed toward carbohydrates and the other toward fat. An α-amylase, called ptyalin, cleaves internal α-1,4-glycosidic bonds present in starch. Exhaustive digestion of starch by this enzyme, which is identical to pancreatic amylase, produces maltose, maltotriose, and α-limit dextrins, which contain the α-1,6 branch points of the original molecule. Salivary amylase has a pH optimum of 7, and it is rapidly denatured at pH 4. However, because a large portion of a meal often remains unmixed for a considerable length of time in the orad stomach, the salivary enzyme may account for the digestion of as much as 75% of the starch present before it is denatured by gastric acid. In the absence of salivary amylase there is no defect in carbohydrate digestion, for the pancreatic enzyme is secreted in amounts sufficient to digest all of the starch present.

The serous salivary glands of the tongue secrete the second digestive enzyme, lingual lipase, which plays a role in the hydrolysis of dietary lipid. Unlike pancreatic lipase its properties allow it to act in all parts of the upper gastrointestinal tract. Thus the ability of lingual lipase to hydrolyze lipids is not affected by surface-active detergents such as bile salts, medium chain fatty acids, and lecithin. It has an acidic pH optimum and remains active through the stomach and into the intestine.

ANATOMY AND INNERVATION OF THE SALIVARY GLANDS

The salivary glands are a collection of somewhat dissimilar structures in the mouth that produce a common juice, the saliva, although the composition of the secretion from different salivary glands differs. The largest of the salivary structures are the paired parotid glands, located near the angle of the jaw and the ear. They secrete a fairly watery juice, whereas the smaller bilateral submandibular and sublingual glands elaborate a more viscid saliva. Other still smaller glands occur in the mucosa covering the palate, buccal areas, lips, and tongue.

Most of the salivary glands are ectodermal in origin. The combined secretion of the parotid and submandibular glands constitutes 90% of the volume of saliva, which in a normal adult amounts to a half liter daily. The specific gravity of this mixed juice ranges from 1.000 to 1.010.

The microscopic structure of the salivary glands combines many features observed in another exocrine gland, the pancreas. A salivary gland consists of a blind-end system of microscopic ducts that branch out from grossly visible ducts. One main duct opens into the mouth from each gland. The functional unit of the salivary duct system, the "salivon," is depicted in Fig. 7-1. At the blind end is the acinus, surrounded by polygonal acinar cells. These cells secrete the initial saliva, including water, electrolytes, and organic molecules such as amylase. Sodium and water follow the chloride. Subsequently the solutes and fluid diffuse out of the acinar cell into the duct lumen to form the initial saliva. The acinar cells are surrounded, in turn, by myoepithelial cells. The myoepithelial cells rest upon the basement membrane of acinar cells. They contain an actinomycin and have motile extensions. The next segment of the salivon is the intercalated duct, which is lined by addi-

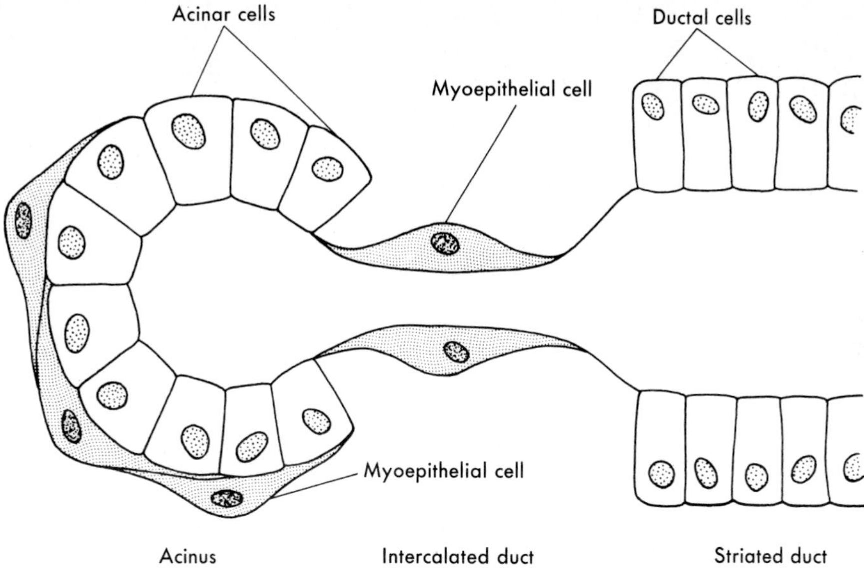

Fig. 7-1. Cells lining the various portions of the salivon.

tional myoepithelial cells. Contraction of myoepithelial cells serves to expel formed saliva from the acinus, oppose retrograde movement of the juice during active secretion of saliva, shorten and widen the internal diameter of the intercalated duct (thereby lowering resistance to the flowing saliva), and prevent distention of the acinum (distention of the blind end of the salivon would permit back-diffusion of formed saliva through the stretched surface of the acinus). Whenever there is an abrupt need for saliva in the mouth, as immediately before vomiting, myoepithelial contraction propels the secretion into the main duct of the gland. Other exocrine glands, such as the mammary glands and the pancreas, also possess myoepithelial cells.

The intercalated duct soon widens to become the striated duct, lined by columnar epithelial cells that resemble the epithelial components of the renal tubule in both shape and function. The saliva in the intercalated duct is similar in ionic composition to plasma. Changes from that composition occur because of ion exchanges in the striated duct. As saliva traverses the striated duct, sodium is actively resorbed from the juice, and potassium is transported into it. Calcium also enters secreting duct cells during salivation. Similarly there is anionic exchange, with chloride being resorbed from the saliva and bicarbonate being added to it.

The striated duct epithelium is considered to be a fairly "tight" sheet membrane; that is, its surface is fairly impermeable to the back-diffusion of water from saliva into tissue, and osmotic gradients can be developed between saliva and interstitial fluid during secretion of potassium into the juice. These osmotic gradients draw water into the saliva from the tissue.

The blood supplied to the salivary glands is distributed by branches of the external carotid artery. The direction of arterial flow within the substance of each salivary gland is opposite the direction of flowing saliva within the ducts of each salivon. The arterioles break up into capillaries around acini and in nonacinar

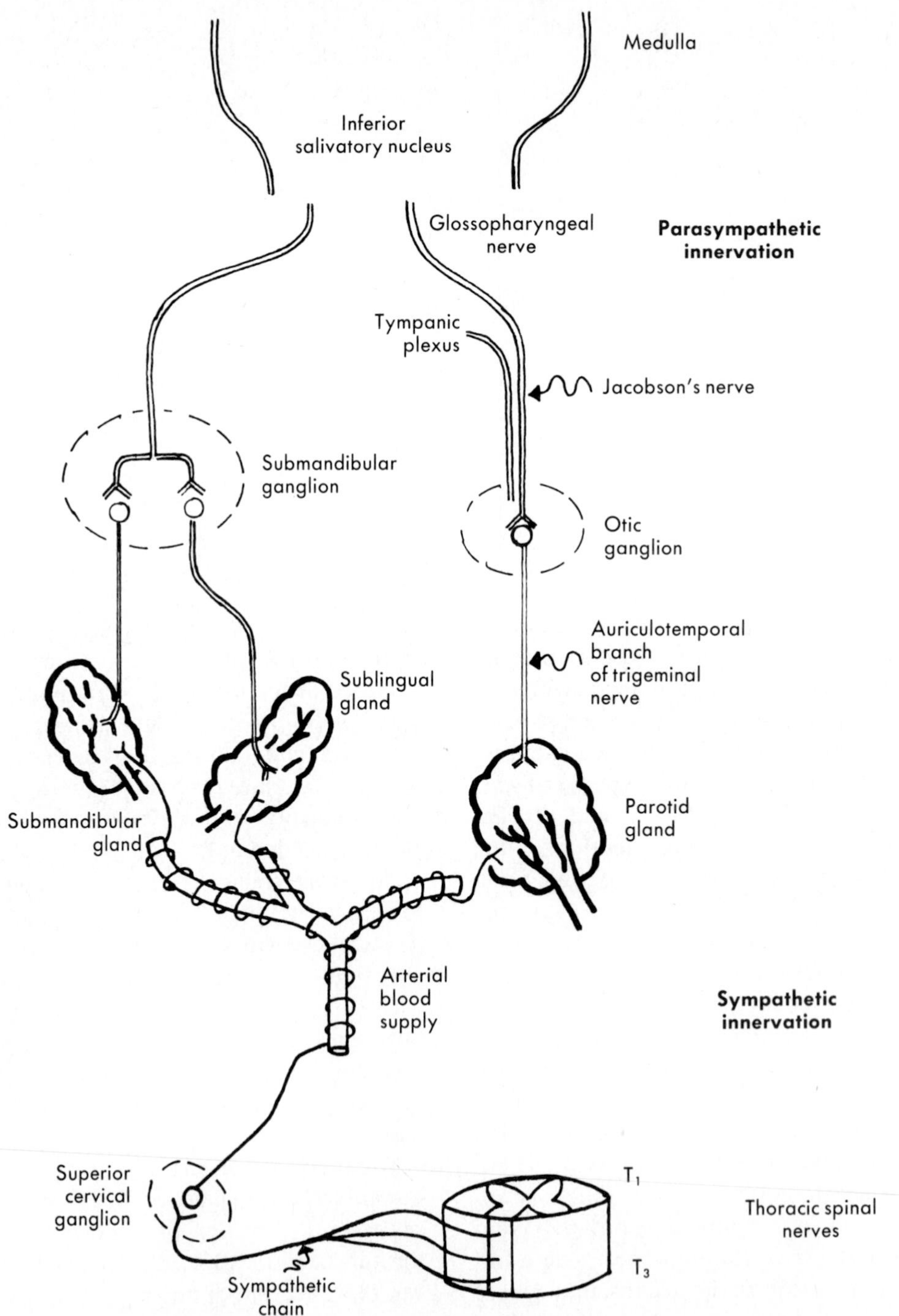

Fig. 7-2. Autonomic nervous distribution to the major salivary glands.

areas as well. Blood from nonacinar areas passes through portal venules back to the acinar capillaries, from which a second set of venules then drains all the blood to the systemic venous circulation. The rate of blood flow through resting salivary tissue is approximately 20 times that through muscle. This in part accounts for the prodigious amounts of saliva produced relative to the weights of the glands.

Both components of the autonomic nervous system reach the salivary glands. The parasympathetic preganglionic fibers are delivered by the facial and glossopharyngeal nerves to autonomic ganglia, from which the postganglionic fibers pass to individual glands. The sympathetic preganglionic nerves originate at the cervical ganglion, whose postganglionic fibers extend to the gland in the periarterial spaces. These relationships appear in Fig. 7-2. Parasympathetic and sympathetic mediators regulate all known salivary gland functions to an extraordinary degree. Their influence includes major effects upon not only secretion but also blood flow, ductular smooth muscle activity, growth, and metabolism of the salivary glands.

COMPOSITION OF SALIVA

The major constituents of saliva are water, electrolytes, and a few enzymes. The unique properties of this gastrointestinal juice are: (1) its large volume relative to the mass of glands that secrete saliva; (2) its low osmolality; (3) its high potassium concentration; and (4) the specific organic materials it contains.

Inorganic Composition

Compared to other secretory organs of the gastrointestinal tract the salivary glands elaborate a remarkably large volume of juice per gram of tissue. Thus, for example, an entire pancreas may reach a maximal rate of secretion of 1 ml/min, whereas at highest rates of secretion in some animals a tiny submaxillary gland can secrete 1 mg/g/min, a fiftyfold higher rate. In humans the salivary glands secrete at rates severalfold higher than other gastrointestinal organs per unit weight of tissue.

The osmolality of saliva is significantly lower than that of plasma at all but the highest rates of secretion, when the saliva becomes isotonic with plasma. As the secretory rate of the salivon increases, the osmolality of its saliva also increases.

The concentrations of electrolytes in saliva vary with the rate of secretion (Fig. 7-3). The potassium concentration of saliva is 2 to 30 times that of the plasma, depending on the rate of secretion, the nature of the stimulus, the plasma potassium concentration, and the level of mineralocorticoids in the circulation. Saliva has the highest potassium concentration of any digestive juice; maximal concentration values approach those within cells. These remarkable levels of salivary potassium imply the existence of an energy-dependent transport mechanism within the salivon. In most species the concentration of Na^+ in saliva is always less than that in plasma, and as the secretory rate increases, the Na^+ concentration also increases. In general, Cl^- concentrations parallel those of Na^+. These findings suggest that Na^+ and Cl^- are secreted and then reabsorbed as the saliva passes through the ducts. The concentration of HCO_3^- in saliva is higher than that in plasma except at low flow rates. This also accounts for the changes in the pH of saliva. At basal rates of flow the pH is slightly acidic but rapidly rises to around 8 as flow is stimulated. The relationships between ion concentrations and flow rates shown in Fig. 7-3 will vary somewhat depending on the stimulus.

The relationships shown in Fig. 7-3 are explained by two basic types of studies that indicate how the final saliva is produced. First, fluid collected by micropuncture of the inter-

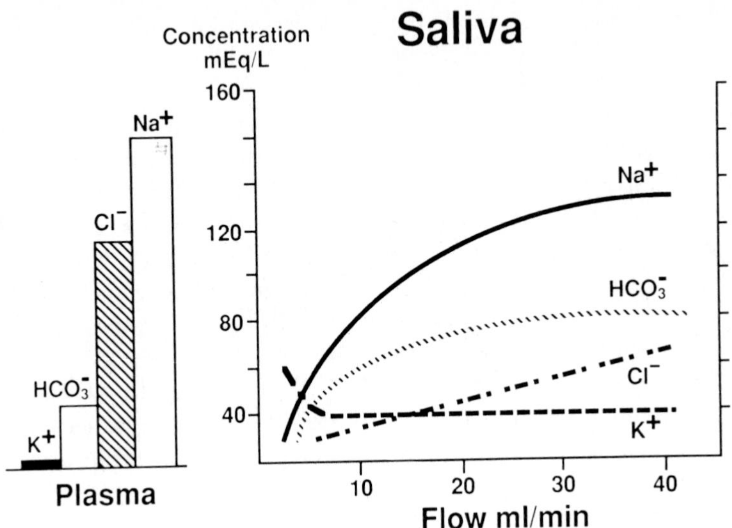

Fig. 7-3. Concentrations of major ions in the saliva as a function of the rate of salivary secretion. Values in plasma are shown for comparison.

calated ducts contains Na, K^+, Cl, and HCO_3 in concentrations approximately equal to their plasma concentrations. This fluid is also isotonic to plasma. Second, if one perfuses a salivary gland duct with fluid containing ions in concentrations similar to those of plasma, Na^+ and Cl^- concentrations are decreased and the K^+ and HCO_3^- concentrations are increased when the fluid is collected at the duct opening. The fluid also becomes hypotonic, and the longer the fluid remains in the duct (i.e., the slower the rate of perfusion) the greater the changes. These data indicate, first, that the acini secrete a fluid similar to plasma in its concentration of ions, and, second, that as the fluid moves down the duct, Na^+ and Cl^- are reabsorbed and K^+ and HCO_3^- are secreted into the saliva. The higher the flow of saliva, the less time is available for modification, and the final saliva more closely resembles plasma in its ionic makeup (Fig. 7-3). At low flow rates K^+ increases considerably and Na^+ and Cl^- decrease. Because most salivary agonists stimulate HCO_3^- secretion, the HCO_3^- concentration remains relatively high even at high rates of secretion. Some K^+ and HCO_3^- are reabsorbed in exchange for Na^+ and Cl^-, but much more Na^+ and Cl^- leave the duct and the saliva becomes hypotonic. Because the duct epithelium is relatively impermeable to water the final product remains hypotonic. These processes are depicted in Fig. 7-4.

Current evidence indicates that Cl^- is the primary ion that is actively secreted by the acinar cells (Fig. 7-5). No evidence exists for direct active secretion of Na^+. The secretory mechanism for Cl^- is inhibited by ouabain, indicating that it depends on the Na^+/K^+ pump in the basolateral membrane. Na^+ moves across the apical membrane of the acinar cell into the lumen, preserving electroneutrality, and water follows down its osmotic gradient. K^+ and HCO_3^- primarily enter saliva passively. Within the ducts, Na^+ is actively absorbed and K^+ actively secreted (Fig. 7-5). Some K^+ is secreted in exchange for H^+. In addition, HCO_3^- is actively secreted in exchange for Cl^-. The net result is a decrease in Na^+ and

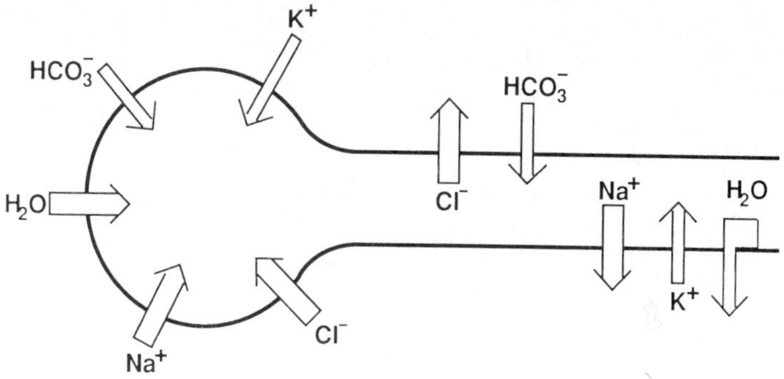

Fig. 7-4. Movements of ions and water in the acinus and duct of the salivon.

Cl^- concentrations and an increase in K^+ and HCO_3^- concentrations and pH as saliva moves down the duct. The active absorption of Na^+ and secretion of K^+ is dependent on the Na^+/K^+ ATPase in the basolateral membrane. Aldosterone acts at the luminal membrane to increase the absorption of Na^+ and secretion of K^+.

Organic Composition

Some organic materials produced and secreted by the salivary glands already have been mentioned in the section describing the functions of saliva. These include the enzymes α-amylase (ptyalin) and lingual lipase, mucus, glycoproteins, lysozymes, and lactoferrin. Another enzyme produced by salivary glands is kallikrein, which converts a plasma protein into the potent vasodilator bradykinin. Kallikrein is released when the metabolism of the salivary glands increases; it is responsible for increased blood flow to the secreting glands. Saliva also contains the blood group substances, A, B, AB, O.

The synthesis of salivary gland enzymes, their storage, and release are similar to the same processes in the pancreas and will be dealt with in Chapter 9. The protein concentration of saliva is about one-tenth the concentration of proteins in the plasma.

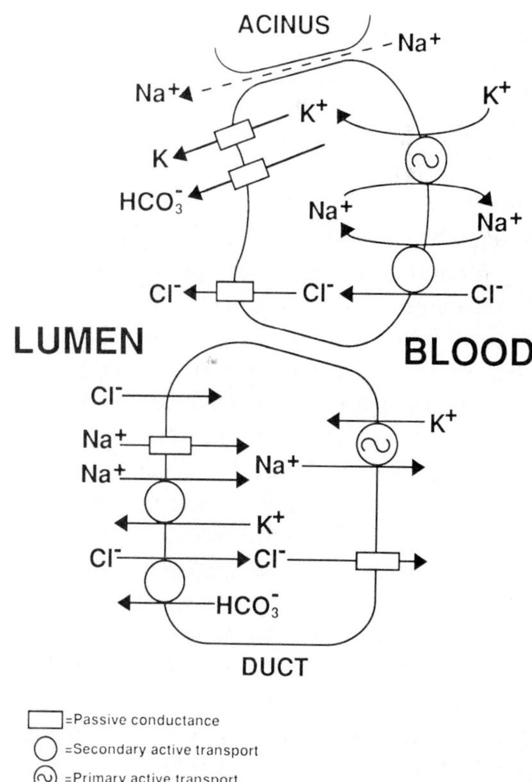

Fig. 7-5. Intracellular mechanisms for the movement of ions in acinar and ductule cells of the salivary glands.

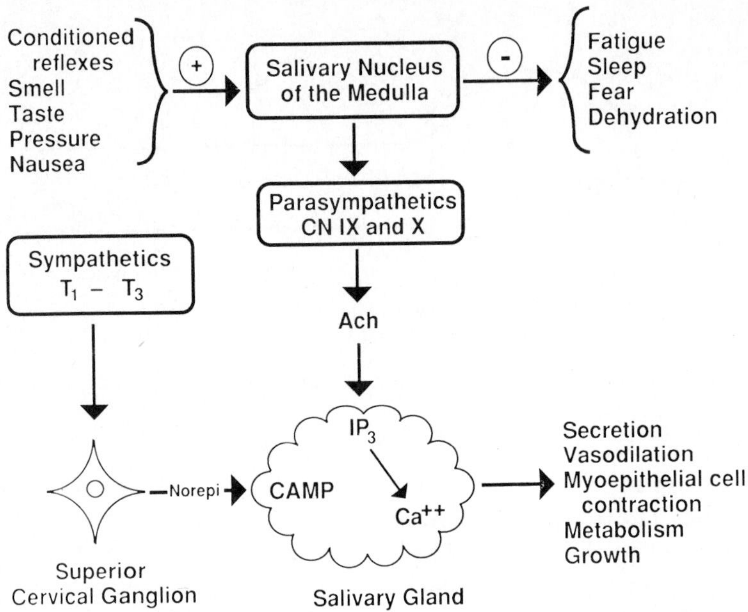

Fig. 7-6. Summary of the regulation of salivary gland function.

REGULATION OF SALIVARY SECRETION

The autonomic nervous system essentially controls all salivary gland secretion. Antidiuretic hormone (ADH, vasopressin) and aldosterone modify the composition of saliva by decreasing its Na^+ concentrations and increasing its K^+ concentrations, but they do not regulate the flow of saliva. The absence of hormonal control of salivation contrasts with the regulation of the flow of gastric and pancreatic juice and bile. The gastrointestinal hormones exert major influences on the secretory activity of the stomach, pancreas, and liver. Control of the salivary glands is also unusual in that both the parasympathetic and sympathetic branches stimulate secretion. The parasympathetic system, however, exerts a much greater influence.

Stimulation of the parasympathetic nerves to the salivary glands begins and maintains salivary secretion. Increased secretion results from the activation of transport processes in both acinar and duct cells. Secretion is enhanced by the contraction of the myoepithelial cells that are innervated by the parasympathetic nerves. Parasympathetic fibers also innervate the surrounding blood vessels, stimulating vasodilation and increasing blood flow to the secreting cells. Increased cellular activity in response to parasympathetic stimulation results in increased consumption of glucose and oxygen and the production of vasodilator metabolites. In addition, kallikrein is released, resulting in the production of the potent vasodilator bradykinin. Increased cellular activity eventually results in growth of the salivary glands. Section of the parasympathetic nerves to the salivary glands causes the glands to atrophy. These processes are outlined in Fig. 7-6.

Sympathetic activation also stimulates secretion, myoepithelial cell contraction, metabolism, and growth of the salivary glands, although these effects are less pronounced and of shorter duration than those produced by the parasympathetics. Stimulation via the sympathetic nerves produces a biphasic change in blood flow to the salivary glands. The earliest response is a decrease caused by activation of α-adrenergic receptors and vasoconstriction. However, as vasodilator metabolites are produced, blood flow increases over resting levels. The effects of sympathetic stimulation also are summarized in Fig. 7-6.

Salivary glands contain receptors to many mediators, but the most important functionally are the muscarinic cholinergic and β-adrenergic receptors. The parasympathetic mediator is acetylcholine, which acts on muscarinic receptors, resulting in the formation of inositol trisphosphate and the subsequent release of Ca^{++} from intracellular stores. Ca^{++} also may enter the cell from outside. The primary sympathetic mediator is norepinephrine, which binds to β-adrenergic receptors resulting in the formation of cAMP. Formation of these second messengers results in protein phosphorylation and enzyme activation that ultimately leads to the stimulation of the salivary glands.

The dual autonomic regulation of the salivary glands is unusual in that the parasympathetic and sympathetic systems both stimulate secretory, metabolic, trophic, muscular, and circulatory functions in similar directions. Their complementary effects are shown in Fig. 7-6.

Ultimately the central nervous system and its autonomic arms are what respond to external events and either stimulate or inhibit activities of the salivary glands. Common events leading to increased glandular activities include chewing, consuming spicy or sour-tasting foods, and smoking. External events leading to glandular inhibition include sleep, fear, dehydration, and fatigue. Glandular activities sensitive to neural control include secretion, circulation, myoepithelial contraction, cellular metabolism, and even parenchymal growth.

Medical events likewise can alter either the amount or the composition of saliva. Besides congenital xerostomia (absence of saliva), there is Sjögren's syndrome, an acquired disease characterized by atrophy of the glands and decreased salivation. The commonly used drugs of the digitalis family cause increased concentrations of calcium and potassium in saliva. In cystic fibrosis, salivary sodium, calcium, and protein are elevated (as are these components in the bronchial secretions, pancreatic juice, and sweat of these patients). Salivary sodium concentrations also are elevated in Addison's disease, though they are decreased in Cushing's syndrome, in primary aldosteronism, and during pregnancy. These electrolytic changes in saliva reflect events or diseases that make similar alterations in other bodily secretions. Excessive salivation is observed with tumors of the mouth or esophagus and with Parkinson's disease. In these cases, unusual local, reflexive, and more general neurological stimuli are responsible.

SUGGESTED REFERENCE

Young JA, Cook DI, van Lennep EW, and Roberts M: Secretion by the major salivary glands. In Johnson LR, editor: Physiology of the gastrointestinal tract, ed 2, New York, 1987, Raven Press.

8 Gastric Secretion

Leonard R. Johnson

Four constituents of gastric juice—intrinsic factor, hydrogen ion, pepsin, and mucus—have physiological functions. They are secreted by the various cells present within the gastric mucosa. The only indispensable ingredient in gastric juice is intrinsic factor, required for the absorption of vitamin B_{12} by the ileal mucosa. Acid is necessary for the conversion of inactive pepsinogen to the enzyme pepsin. Acid and pepsin begin the digestion of protein, but in their absence pancreatic enzymes hydrolyze all ingested protein, so no nitrogen is wasted in the stools. Acid also kills a large number of bacteria that enter the stomach, thereby reducing the number of organisms reaching the intestine. In cases of severely reduced or absent acid secretion the incidence of intestinal infections is greater. Mucus lines the wall of the stomach, protecting it from damage. It acts primarily as a lubricant, protecting the mucosa from physical injury. It neutralizes a small amount of acid, though it is not the major factor responsible for the normal stomach's resistance to acid and peptic digestion.

Gastric juice and many of its functions originally were described by a young army surgeon, William Beaumont, stationed at a fort on Mackinac Island in northern Michigan. Beaumont was called to treat a French Canadian, Alexis St. Martin, who had been shot accidentally in the side at close range with a shotgun. St. Martin unexpectedly survived but was left with a permanent opening into his stomach from the outside (gastric fistula). The accident occurred in 1822, and during the ensuing 3 years Beaumont nursed St. Martin back to health. Beaumont retained St. Martin "for the purpose of making physiological experiments," which were begun in 1825. Beaumont's observations and conclusions, many of which remain unchanged today, included a description of the juice itself and its digestive and bacteriostatic functions, the identification of the acid as hydrochloric, the realization that mucus was a separate secretion, the realization that mental disturbances affected gastric function, a direct study of gastric motility, and a thorough study of the ability of gastric juices to digest various foodstuffs.

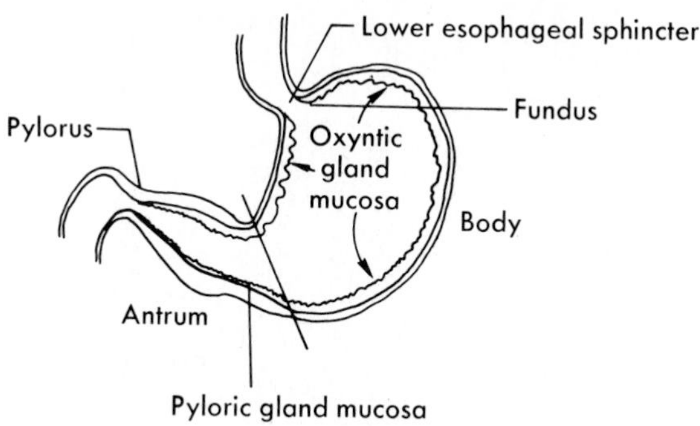

Fig. 8-1. Areas of the stomach.

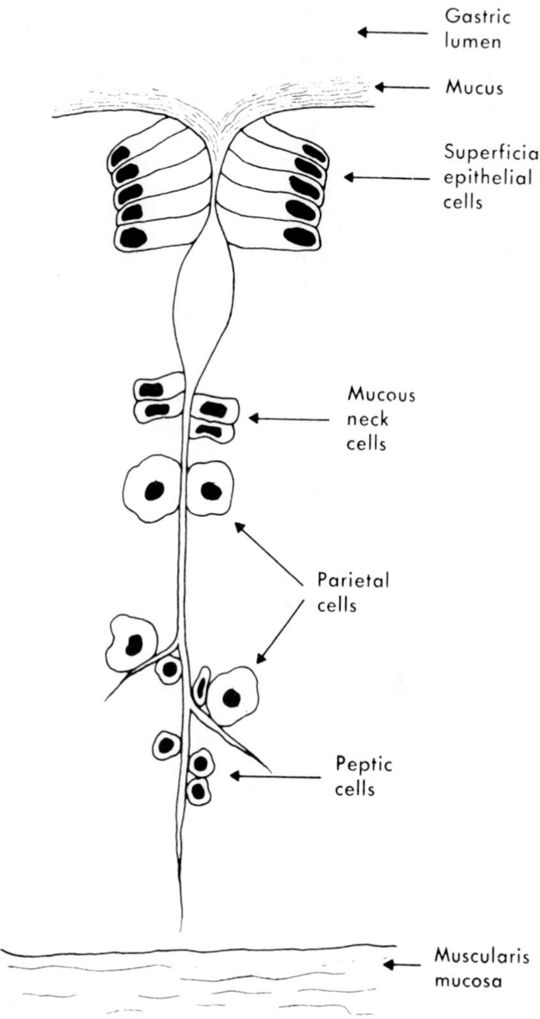

Fig. 8-2. Oxyntic gland and surface pit. Note the positions of the various cell types.

FUNCTIONAL ANATOMY

Functionally the gastric mucosa is divided into the oxyntic gland area and the pyloric gland area (Fig. 8-1). The oxyntic gland mucosa secretes acid and is located in the proximal 80% of the stomach. It includes the body and the fundus. The distal 20% of the gastric mucosa, referred to as the pyloric gland mucosa, synthesizes and releases the hormone gastrin. This area of the stomach often is designated as the "antrum."

The gastric mucosa is composed of pits and glands (Fig. 8-2). The pits and surface itself are lined with mucous or surface epithelial cells. At the base of the pits are the openings of the glands, which project into the mucosa toward the outside or serosa. The oxyntic glands contain the acid-producing parietal cells and the peptic or chief cells, which secrete the enzyme precursor pepsinogen. Pyloric glands contain the gastrin-producing G cells and mucous cells, which also produce pepsinogen. Mucous neck cells are present where the glands open into the pits. These cells divide, and the daughter cells migrate both to the surface, where they differentiate into mucous cells, and down into the glands, where they become parietal cells in the oxyntic gland area. Endocrine cells such as the G cells also differentiate from mucous neck cells. Peptic cells are capable of mitosis, but there is evidence that they also can arise from mucous neck cells during the repair of damage to the mucosa. Cells of the surface and pits are replaced much more rapidly than are those of the glands.

The parietal cells secrete hydrochloric acid and, in humans, intrinsic factor. In some species the chief cells secrete intrinsic factor.

A

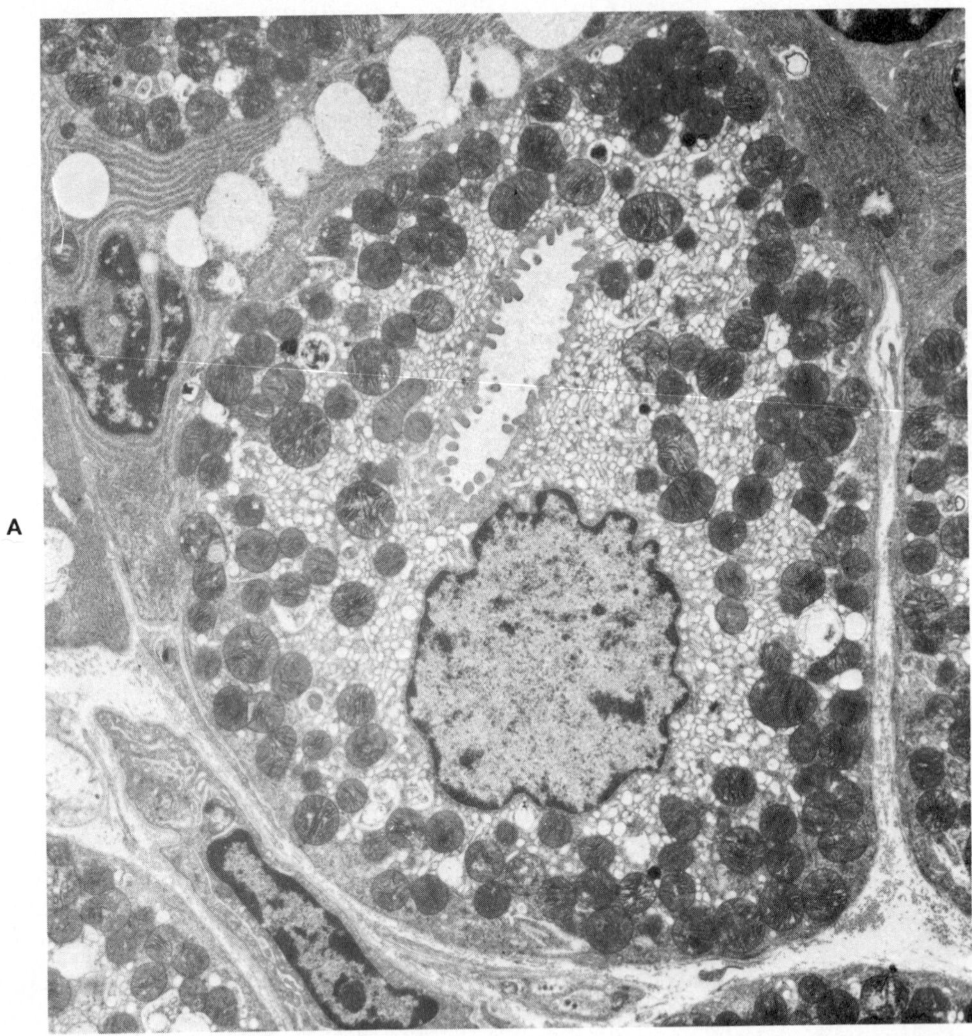

Fig. 8-3. Parietal cell. **A**, Electron photomicrograph. *(A, Courtesy Dr. Bruce MacKay.)*
Continued.

The normal human stomach contains approximately one billion parietal cells, which produce acid at a concentration of 150 to 160 mEq/L. The human stomach secretes 1 to 2 L of gastric juice per day. Because the pH of the final juice at high rates of secretion may be less than 1 and that of the blood is 7.4, the parietal cells must expend a large amount of energy to concentrate hydrogen ions. The energy for the production of this more than a millionfold concentration gradient comes from ATP produced by the numerous mitochondria located within the cell (Fig. 8-3).

During the resting state the cytoplasm of the parietal cells is dominated by numerous tubulovesicles. There is also an intracellular canaliculus that is continuous with the lumen of the oxyntic gland. After stimulation of acid

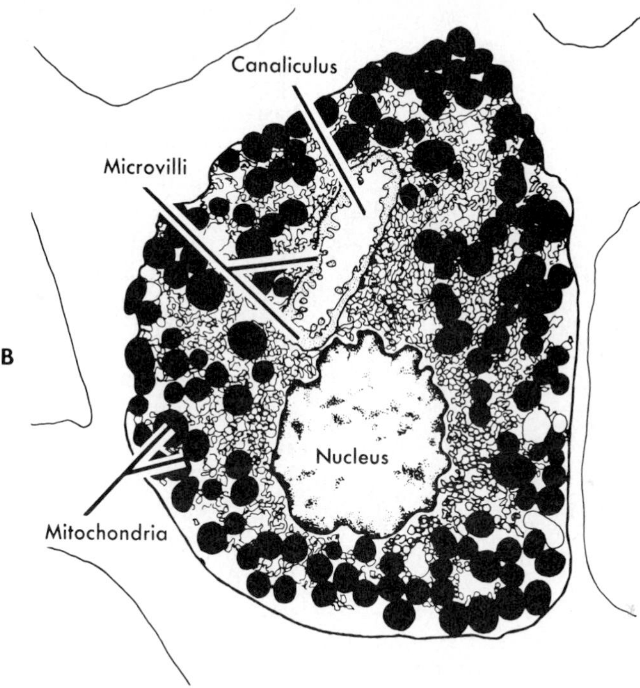

Fig. 8-3, cont'd. **B,** Schematic.

secretion the tubulovesicles become microvilli and project into the canaliculus, which has become greatly expanded to occupy much of the cell. Carbonic anhydrase and ATPase, enzymes necessary for the production and secretion of acid, are localized in the microvilli. The activities of these enzymes increase during acid secretion. Acid secretion begins within 10 minutes of administering a stimulant. This lag time probably is expended in the morphological conversion and enzyme activations described previously.

The surface epithelial mucous cells are recognized primarily by the large number of mucous granules at their apical surfaces. During secretion the membranes of the granules fuse with the cell membrane, expelling mucus.

Peptic cells contain a highly developed endoplasmic reticulum for the synthesis of pepsinogen. The proenzyme is packaged into zymogen granules by the numerous Golgi structures within the cytoplasm. The zymogen granules migrate to the apical surface, where during secretion they empty their contents into the lumen by exocytosis. This entire procedure of enzyme synthesis, packaging, and secretion is discussed in greater detail in Chapter 9.

Endocrine cells of the gut also contain numerous granules. However, unlike the peptic and mucous cells, these hormone-containing granules are located at the base of the cell. The hormones are secreted into the intercellular space, from which they diffuse into the capillaries. The endocrine cells have numerous microvilli extending from their apical surface into the lumen. Presumably the microvilli contain receptors that sample the luminal

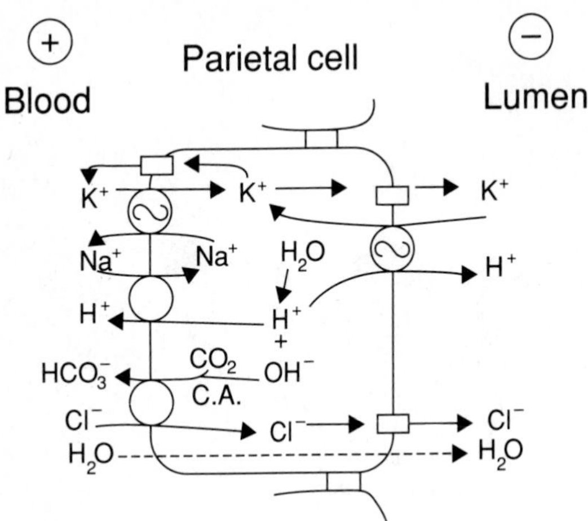

Fig. 8-4. Transport processes in the gastric mucosa accounting for the presence of the various ions in gastric juice and for the negative transmembrane potential.

contents and trigger hormone secretion in response to the appropriate stimuli.

SECRETION OF ACID

The transport processes involved in the secretion of hydrochloric acid are shown in Fig. 8-4. The exact biochemical steps for the production of H^+ are not known, but the reaction can be summarized as:

$$HOH \rightarrow OH^- + H^+ \quad (1)$$

$$OH^- + CO_2 \xrightarrow{CA} HCO_3^- \quad (2)$$

H^+ is pumped actively into the lumen and HCO_3^- diffuses into the blood, giving gastric venous blood a higher pH than arterial blood when the stomach is secreting. Step 2 is catalyzed by carbonic anhydrase. Inhibition of this enzyme decreases the rate but does not prevent acid secretion. Metabolism produces much of the CO_2 used to neutralize OH^-, but at high secretory rates CO_2 from the blood also is required. The active transport of H^+ across the mucosal membrane is catalyzed by H^+, K^+-ATPase, and H^+ is pumped into the lumen in exchange for K^+. Within the cell, K^+ is accumulated by the Na^+-K^+-ATPase in the basolateral membrane. Accumulated K^+ moves down its electrochemical gradient, leaking across both membranes. Luminal K^+ is therefore recycled by the H^+-K^+-ATPase. Cl^- enters the cell across the basolateral membrane in exchange for HCO_3^-. The pumping of H^+ out of the cell allows OH^- to accumulate and form HCO_3^- from CO_2, a step catalyzed by carbonic anhydrase. The HCO_3^- entering the blood causes its pH to increase, so the gastric venous blood from the actively secreting stomach has a higher pH than arterial blood. The production of OH^- is facilitated by the low intracellular Na^+ concentration established by the Na^+-K^+-ATPase. Some Na^+ moves down its gradient back into the cell in exchange for H^+, further increasing OH^- production. This in turn increases HCO_3^- production, enhancing the driving force for the entry of Cl^- and its uphill movement from the blood into the lumen. Thus the movement of Cl^- from blood to lumen against both electrical and chemical gradients is the result of excess OH^- in the cell after the H^+ has been pumped out.

ORIGIN OF THE ELECTRICAL POTENTIAL DIFFERENCE

The potential difference across the resting oxyntic gland mucosa is -70 to -80 mV lumen negative with respect to the blood. This charge separation primarily is caused by the secretion of Cl^- (see previous section) against its electrochemical gradient. This is accomplished by both surface epithelial cells and parietal cells. Following the stimulation of acid secretion the potential difference decreases to -30 or -40 mV because the positively changed H^+ moves in the same direction as Cl^-. H^+, therefore, actually is secreted

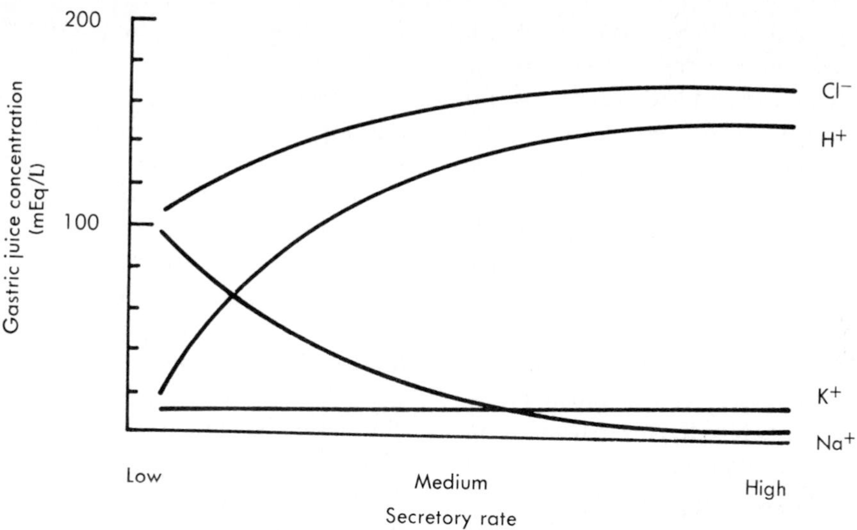

Fig. 8-5. Relationship of the electrolyte concentrations in gastric juice to the rate of gastric secretion.

down its electrical gradient, facilitating its transport against a several millionfold concentration gradient.

To produce an electrical gradient and a millionfold concentration gradient of H^+ there must be minimal leakage of ions and acid back into the mucosa. The ability of the stomach to prevent leakage is attributed to the so-called gastric mucosal barrier. If this barrier is disrupted by aspirin, alcohol, bile, or a number of agents that damage the gastric mucosa, the potential difference decreases as ions leak down their electrochemical gradients. The exact nature of the barrier is unknown; its properties and the consequences of disrupting it are discussed more fully in the section on the pathophysiology of ulcer diseases (p. 81). The negative potential difference across the stomach facilitates acid secretion because H^+ is secreted down the electrical gradient. The potential difference can be used to position catheters within the digestive tract. With an electrode placed at the catheter tip the oxyntic gland mucosa can be distinguished readily from the esophagus (potential difference, −15 mV) or the duodenum (potential difference, −5 mV).

ELECTROLYTES OF GASTRIC JUICE

The concentrations of the major electrolytes in gastric juice are variable but usually are related to the rate of secretion (Fig. 8-5). At low rates the final juice is essentially a solution of NaCl with small amounts of H^+ and K^+. As the rate increases the concentration of Na^+ decreases and that of H^+ increases. The concentrations of both Cl^- and K^+ rise slightly as the secretory rate rises. At peak rates, gastric juice is primarily HCl with small amounts of Na^+ and K^+. At all rates of secretion the concentrations of H^+, K^+, and Cl^- are higher than those in plasma, and the concentration of Na^+ is lower than that in plasma. Thus gastric juice and plasma—regardless of the secretory rate—are approximately isotonic.

To help understand the changes in ionic concentration it is convenient to think of gastric juice as a mixture of two separate secretions: a nonparietal and a parietal component. The nonparietal component is a basal alkaline secretion of constant and low volume. Its primary constituents are Na^+ and Cl^-, and it contains K^+ at about the same concentration as does plasma. In the absence of H^+ secretion, HCO_3^- can be detected in gastric juice. The HCO_3^- is secreted at a concentration of about 30 mEq/L. The nonparietal component is always present, and the parietal component is secreted against this background. As the rate of secretion increases, and because the increase is caused solely by the parietal component, the concentrations of electrolytes in the final juice begin to approach those of pure parietal cell secretion. Pure parietal cell secretion is slightly hyperosmotic and contains 150 to 160 mEq H^+/L and 10 to 20 mEq K^+/L. The only anion present is Cl^-.

This so-called two-component model of gastric secretion is an oversimplification. Parietal secretion is modified somewhat by the exchange of Na^+ for H^+ as the juice moves up the gland into the lumen. Although such changes are minimal they do participate in determining the final ionic composition of gastric juice.

A knowledge of the composition of gastric juice is required to treat a patient with chronic vomiting or one whose gastric juice is being aspirated and who is being maintained intravenously. Replacement of only NaCl and dextrose will result in hypokalemic metabolic alkalosis, which can be fatal.

STIMULANTS OF ACID SECRETION

Only a few agents directly stimulate the parietal cells to secrete acid. The antral hormone gastrin and the parasympathetic mediator acetylcholine are the most important physiological regulators. In fact, gastrin is the most effective gastric secretagogue known and on a molar basis is 1500 times more potent than histamine. Acetylcholine stimulates gastrin release in addition to stimulating the parietal cell directly.

Evidence has accumulated that an unknown hormone of intestinal origin also stimulates acid secretion. This substance tentatively has been named *enterooxyntin* to denote both its origin and its action. In humans, circulating amino acids also stimulate the parietal cell and provide some of the stimulation of acid secretion that results from the presence of food in the small intestine.

Histamine, which occurs in many tissues (including the entire gastrointestinal tract), is a potent stimulator of parietal cell secretion. There is little evidence that histamine release is regulated in most mammals and that it in turn regulates acid secretion in the sense that gastrin and acetylcholine do. It nevertheless plays an essential role in the stimulation of gastric secretion.

ROLE OF HISTAMINE IN ACID SECRETION

In 1920 a Polish physiologist, Popielski, discovered that histamine stimulated gastric acid secretion. It was then believed by many that gastrin was actually histamine. The confusion cleared somewhat in 1938 when Komarov demonstrated that there were two separate secretagogues in the gastric mucosa. He showed that trichloroacetic acid precipitated the peptide gastrin from gastric mucosal extracts, leaving histamine in the supernatant. It was then suggested by MacIntosh that histamine was the final common mediator of acid secretion. He proposed that gastrin and acetylcholine released histamine, which in turn stimulated the parietal cells directly and was the only direct stimulant of the parietal cells.

At this point it is important to introduce and define the concept of "potentiation." Potentiation is said to occur between two stimulants if the response to their simultaneous administration exceeds the sum of the responses when each is administered alone. A number of secretory responses in the gastrointestinal tract depend on the potentiation of two or more agonists. In the stomach histamine potentiates the effects of gastrin and acetylcholine on the parietal cell. Acetylcholine also potentiates the response to gastrin. In this way small amounts of stimuli acting together often can produce a near-maximal secretory response. Potentiation requires the presence of separate receptors on the target cell for each stimulant and, in the case of acid secretion, is incompatible with the final common mediator hypothesis.

Until recently all antihistamines blocked only the histamine H_1-receptor, which mediates actions such as bronchoconstriction and vasodilation. The stimulation of acid secretion by histamine is mediated by the H_2-receptor and is not blocked by conventional antihistamines. A new H_2-receptor antagonist, cimetidine, effectively inhibits histamine-stimulated acid secretion. Cimetidine, however, has been found also to inhibit the secretory responses to gastrin, acetylcholine, and food. Atropine, a specific antagonist of the muscarinic actions of acetylcholine, blocks the acid responses to gastrin and histamine as well as to acetylcholine. When preparations of isolated parietal cells (which rule out the presence of stimuli other than those directly added) are used, it has been shown that the effects of cimetidine on gastrin- and acetylcholine-stimulated secretion are caused by the inhibition of the part of the secretory response resulting from histamine potentiation. Similarly the inhibition of gastrin- and histamine-stimulated secretion by atropine is caused by removal of the potentiating effects of acetylcholine. It is assumed that histamine is present in background concentrations. There is no evidence in humans that the amount of histamine acting on the parietal cell increases during the stimulation of acid secretion.

A model based on these results is shown in

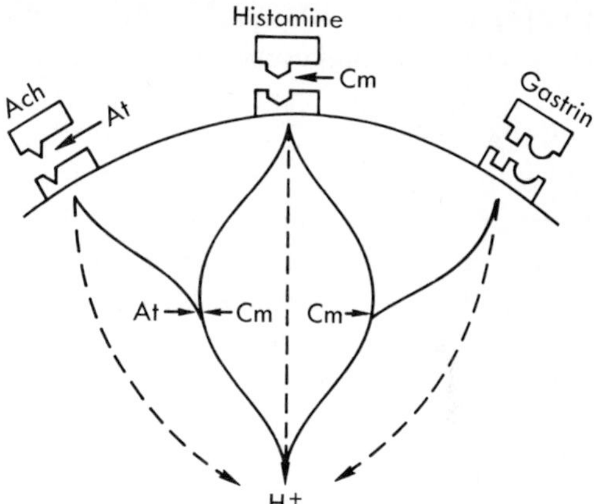

Fig. 8-6. Interactions of histamine, gastrin, and acetylcholine on the parietal cell membrane. *(Adapted from Soll AH: J Clin Invest 61:381-389, 1968.)*

Fig. 8-6. There are separate receptors for acetylcholine, histamine, and gastrin on the parietal cell membrane. Potentiated stimulation is depicted by solid arrows, and direct effects of the secretagogues by broken arrows. Responses blocked by cimetidine are indicated by *Cm*, and those blocked by atropine by *At*. Cimetidine is a more effective inhibitor of acid secretion than atropine and has fewer side effects. It is an extremely effective drug for the treatment of duodenal ulcer disease.

STIMULATION OF ACID SECRETION

The unstimulated human stomach secretes acid at a rate equal to 10% to 15% of that present during maximal stimulation. The stomach emptied of food therefore contains a relatively small volume of gastric juice. The pH of this fluid is usually less than 2.0. Thus in the absence of food the gastric mucosa is acidified.

The stimulation of gastric secretion is conveniently divided into three phases based on the location of the receptors initiating the secretory responses. It is important to realize that this division is artificial; shortly after the start of a meal, stimulation is initiated from all three areas at the same time.

Cephalic Phase

Chemoreceptors and mechanoreceptors located in the tongue and the buccal and nasal cavities are stimulated by tasting, smelling, chewing, and swallowing food. The afferent nerve impulses are relayed through the vagal nucleus and vagal efferent fibers to the stomach. Even the thought of an appetizing meal stimulates gastric secretion. The secretory response to cephalic stimulation depends greatly on the nature of the meal. The greatest response occurs to an appetizing self-selected meal. A bland meal produces a much smaller response. The efferent pathway for the cephalic phase is the vagus nerve. The entire response is blocked by vagotomy.

The cephalic phase is best studied by the procedure known as sham-feeding. A dog is prepared with esophageal and gastric fistulas. When the esophageal fistula is open, swallowed food falls to the exterior without entering the stomach. Gastric secretion is collected from the gastric fistula, and its volume and acid content are measured. Stimulation during the cephalic phase represents about 30% of the total response to a meal. The cephalic phase also can be studied using a variety of drugs. Hypoglycemia introduced by tolbutamide or insulin, or interference with glucose metabolism by glucose analogues such as 3-methylglucose or 2-deoxyglucose, activates hypothalamic centers that stimulate secretion via the vagus nerve.

The vagus acts directly on the parietal cells to stimulate acid secretion. It also acts upon the antral gastrin cells to stimulate gastrin release. The mediator at the parietal cells is acetylcholine. The mediator at the gastrin cell is GRP (gastrin-releasing peptide or bombesin). The direct effect on the parietal cell is the more important in humans, for selective vagotomy of the parietal cell–containing area of the stomach abolishes the response to sham-feeding, whereas antrectomy only moderately reduces it. The complete inhibition of the response to sham-feeding caused by vagotomy is partly caused by the elimination of the potentiated response between acetylcholine and gastrin. The mechanisms involved in the cephalic phase are illustrated in Fig. 8-7.

Gastric Phase

When swallowed food first enters the stomach and mixes with the small volume of juice normally present, buffers (primarily protein) contained in the food neutralize the acid. The pH of the gastric contents may rise to 6 or above. Because gastrin release is inhibited when the antral pH drops below 3 and is prevented totally when the pH is less than 2, essentially no gastrin is released from the stomach that is void of food. The rise in pH permits vagal stimulation from the cephalic phase to initiate, and stimuli from the gastric phase to maintain, gastrin release. It is important to realize that increasing the pH of the gastric contents is not, in itself, a stimulus for gastrin release but merely allows other stimuli to be effective.

Distention of the stomach and bathing the gastric mucosa with certain chemicals, primarily amino acids and peptides, are the effective stimuli of the gastric phase. Distention activates mechanoreceptors in the mucosa of both the oxyntic and the pyloric gland areas. It also may activate long extramural reflexes or local short intramural reflexes. All distention reflexes are mediated cholinergically and can be blocked by atropine.

Long reflexes also are called vagovagal reflexes, meaning that both afferent impulses and efferent impulses are carried by neurons in the vagus nerve. Mucosal distention receptors send signals by vagal afferents to the vagal nucleus. Efferent signals are sent back to G

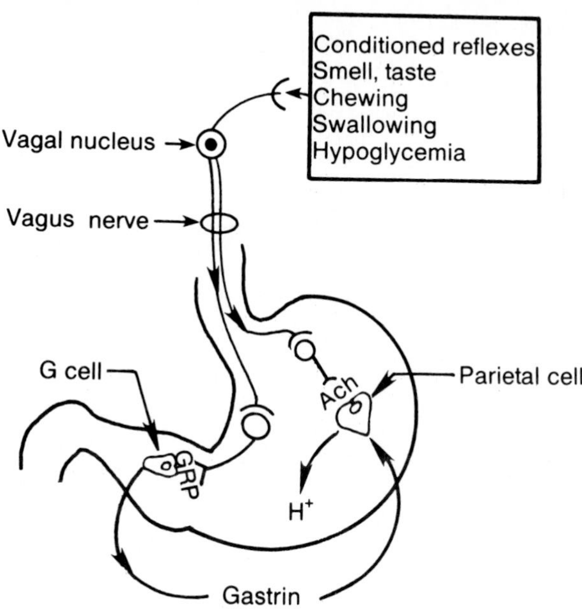

Fig. 8-7. Mechanisms stimulating gastric acid secretion during the cephalic phase.

cells and parietal cells by the vagal efferents.

Short or local reflexes are mediated by neurons that are contained entirely within the wall of the stomach. These may be single-neuron reflexes, or they may involve intermediary neurons. There are two local distention reflexes. Both of these are regional reflexes, meaning that the receptor and effector are located in the same area of the stomach. Distention of a vagally innervated pyloric (antrum) pouch stimulates gastrin release. The effect is decreased, but not abolished, by vagotomy—meaning that the gastrin response is mediated by both vagovagal reflexes and local reflexes. This local reflex is called a pyloropyloric reflex.

Distention of an antral pouch with pH 1 hydrochloric acid stimulates acid secretion from the oxyntic gland area. Because gastrin release does not take place when the pH is below 2, the increase in acid output must be mediated by a neural reflex. As the discerning reader will have surmised, this vagovagal reflex is known as a "pylorooxyntic reflex." Distention reflexes, which are much more effective stimulants of the parietal cell than they are of the G cell, are illustrated diagrammatically in Fig. 8-8.

Peptides and amino acids stimulate gastrin release from the G cells. This effect is not blocked by vagotomy. Only part of it appears to be blocked by atropine, indicating that protein digestion products contain chemicals capable of directly stimulating the G cell to release gastrin. Acidification of the antral mucosa below pH 3 inhibits gastrin release in response to digested protein. A few other commonly ingested substances are also capable of stimulating acid secretion. Caffeine stimulates the parietal cells directly. Calcium, either in the gastric lumen or as elevated serum concentrations, stimulates gastrin release and acid secretion. Considerable debate exists about the effects of alcohol on gastric secretion. Alcohol has been shown to stimulate gastrin release and acid secretion in some

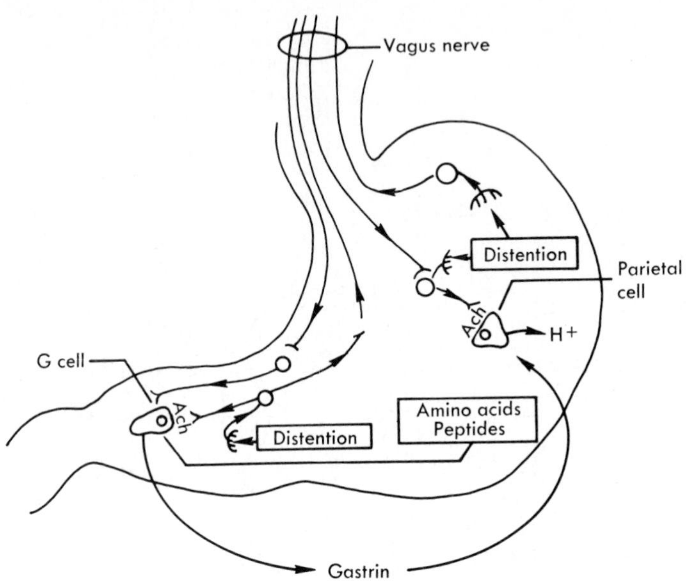

Fig. 8-8. Mechanisms stimulating gastric acid secretion during the gastric phase.

species; however, these effects do not appear to take place in humans.

Release of Gastrin

Considerable evidence has accumulated favoring a mechanism similar to that in Fig. 8-9 to explain the regulation of gastrin release. GRP acts on the G cell to stimulate gastrin release, and somatostatin acts on the G cell to inhibit release. GRP is a neurocrine released by vagal stimulation. This explains why atropine does not block vagally mediated gastrin release. Somatostatin acts as a paracrine and its release is inhibited by vagal stimulation. In the isolated, perfused rat stomach, vagal stimulation increases GRP release and decreases somatostatin release into the perfusate. Thus it appears that vagal activation stimulates gastrin by releasing GRP and by inhibiting the release of somatostatin. Acid in the lumen of the stomach is believed to act directly on the somatostatin cell to stimulate the release of somatostatin, thereby preventing gastrin release. Protein digestion products, especially amines, may act directly on the G cell (or be absorbed by the G cell) to stimulate gastrin release.

There are data indicating that atropine can block some gastrin release stimulated by protein digestion products. This is evidence that luminal receptors may be activated, resulting in a cholinergic reflex that leads to gastrin release. There is also evidence that this reflex may operate by releasing GRP and inhibiting somatostatin release. Much of the foregoing is not proved, but the student should be familiar with the major components of this mechanism.

Intestinal Phase

Protein digestion products in the duodenum stimulate acid secretion from denervated gastric mucosa, indicating the presence of a hormonal mechanism. In humans the proximal duodenum is rich in gastrin, which has been shown to contribute to the serum gastrin response to a meal. In dogs, liver extract re-

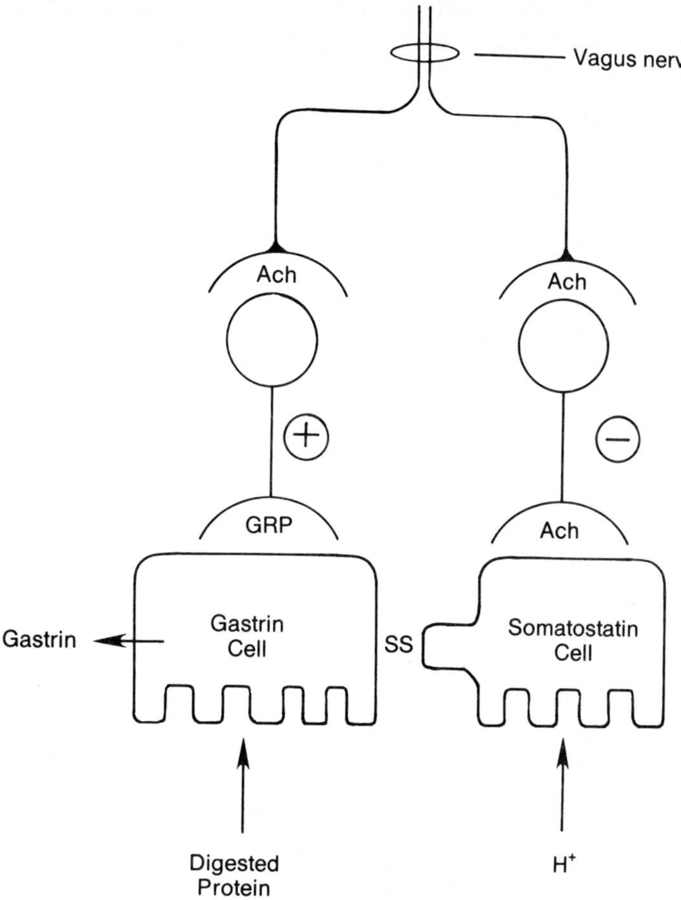

Fig. 8-9. Mechanism for the regulation of gastrin release.

leases a hormone from the duodenal mucosa that stimulates acid secretion without increasing serum gastrin levels. This hormone tentatively has been named "enterooxyntin." Its significance in humans is unknown.

Intravenous infusion of amino acids has recently been shown to stimulate acid secretion. Therefore a good portion of the stimulation attributed to the intestinal phase may be caused by absorbed amino acids. Intestinal stimuli result in much less acid secretion than do stimuli from either the cephalic or the gastric phases. The gastric phase is responsible for most acid secretion.

Fig. 8-10 summarizes the mechanisms and final stimulants acting in all three phases.

INHIBITION OF ACID SECRETION

When food first enters the stomach, its buffers neutralize the small volume of gastric acid present during the interdigestive phase. As the pH of the antral mucosa rises above 3, gastrin is released by the stimuli of the cephalic and gastric phases. One hour after the meal the rate of gastric secretion is maximal, the buffering capacity of the meal is saturated, a significant portion of the meal has emptied from the stomach, and the acid concentration

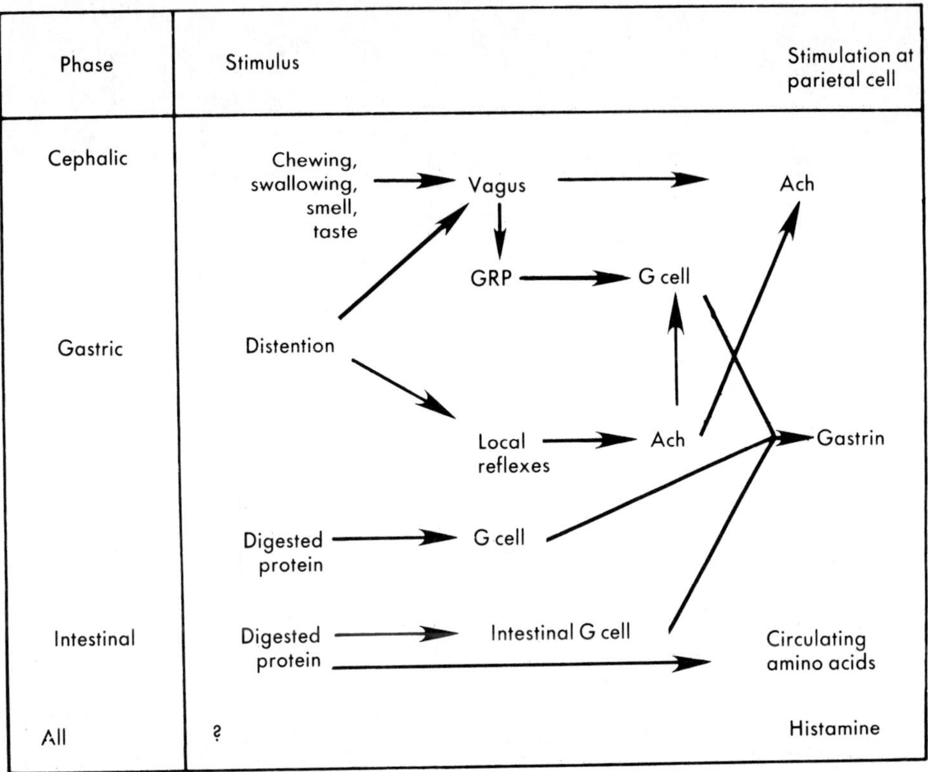

Fig. 8-10. Mechanisms for stimulating acid secretion.

of the gastric contents increases. As the pH falls, gastrin release is inhibited, removing a significant factor for the stimulation of gastric acid secretion. This passive negative feedback mechanism is extremely important in the regulation of acid secretion. In addition somatostatin released by the drop in intragastric pH also directly inhibits the parietal cells.

Evidence exists for several hormonal mechanisms for the active inhibition of gastric acid secretion. These hormones are released from duodenal mucosa by acid, fatty acids, or hyperosmotic solutions and collectively are termed "enterogastrones." They often inhibit gastric emptying as well as acid secretion. Teleologically these mechanisms ensure that the gastric contents are delivered to the small bowel at a rate that does not exceed the capacity for digestion and absorption. They also prevent damage to the duodenal mucosa that can result from acidic and hyperosmotic solutions.

GIP is released by fatty acids and acts at the parietal cell to inhibit acid secretion. Secretin also may be classified as an enterogastrone because it also inhibits gastric acid secretion. The importance and physiological significance of these effects in humans have not been determined. CCK is a physiologically significant inhibitor of gastric emptying. Hyperosmotic solutions release an as yet unidentified enterogastrone. Strong evidence also exists that acid initiates a nervous reflex from receptors in the duodenal mucosa that suppresses acid secretion. These mechanisms are summarized in Fig. 8-11.

Region	Stimulus	Mediator	Inhibit gastrin release	Inhibit acid secretion
Antrum	Acid (pH < 3.0)	Somatostatin	+	+
Duodenum	Acid	Secretin	+	+
		Nervous reflex		+
	Hyperosmotic solutions	Unidentified enterogastrone		+
Duodenum and jejunum	Fatty acids	GIP	+	+
		Unidentified enterogastrone		+

Fig. 8-11. Mechanisms for inhibiting acid secretion.

PEPSIN

Pepsinogen has a molecular weight of 42,500 and is split to form the active enzyme pepsin, which has a molecular weight of 35,000. Pepsinogen is converted to pepsin in the gastric juice when the pH drops below 5. Pepsin itself can catalyze the formation of additional pepsin from pepsinogen. Pepsin begins the digestion of protein by splitting interior peptide linkages (see Chapter 11).

Pepsinogens belong to two main groups, I and II. Those in the first group are secreted by peptic and mucous cells of the oxyntic glands; those in the second, by mucous cells present in the pyloric gland area and duodenum as well as in the oxyntic gland area. Pepsinogens appear in the blood, and there is considerable evidence that their levels may be correlated with duodenal ulcer formation. This is discussed in connection with peptic ulcer disease (p. 83).

The strongest stimulant of pepsinogen secretion is acetylcholine. Thus vagal activation during both cephalic and gastric phases results in a significant proportion of the total pepsinogen secreted. Hydrogen ion plays an important role in several areas of pepsin physiology. First, acid is necessary to convert pepsinogen to the active enzyme pepsin. At pH 2 this conversion is almost instantaneous. Second, acid triggers a local cholinergic reflex that stimulates the chief cells to secrete. This mechanism is atropine sensitive and may account in part for the strong correlation between acid and pepsin outputs. Third, the acid-sensitive reflex greatly enhances the effects of other stimuli on the peptic cell. This mechanism ensures that large amounts of pepsinogen are not secreted unless sufficient acid for conversion to pepsin is present. Fourth, acid releases the hormone secretin from duodenal mucosa. Secretin also stimulates pepsinogen secretion, although it is questionable whether enough secretin is present to do so under normal conditions.

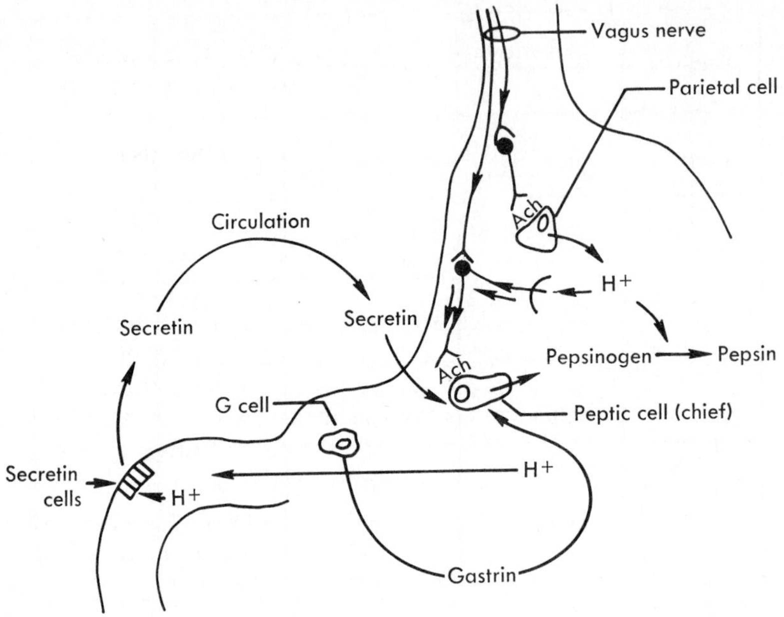

Fig. 8-12. Summary for mechanisms for stimulating pepsinogen secretion and activation to pepsin.

The hormone gastrin usually is listed as a pepsigogue. Infusion of gastrin increases pepsin secretion. In dogs the entire response can be accounted for by the stimulation of acid secretion by gastrin and the subsequent activation of the acid-sensitive reflex mechanism for pepsinogen secretion. In humans gastrin may be a weak pepsigogue in its own right. The mechanisms regulating pepsinogen secretion are summarized in Fig. 8-12.

MUCUS

Vagal nerve stimulation and acetylcholine increase soluble mucus secretion from the mucous neck cells. Soluble mucus consists of mucoproteins and mixes with the gastric chyme lubricating it.

Surface mucous cells secrete visible or insoluble mucus in response to chemical stimulants (such as ethanol) and in response to physical contact and friction with roughage in the diet. Visible mucus is secreted as a gel that entraps the alkaline component of the surface cell secretion. It is present during the interdigestive phase and protects the mucosa with an alkaline layer of lubricant. A portion of this coating is made up of mucus-containing surface cells that have been shed and trapped in the layer of mucus. During the response to a meal, insoluble mucus protects the mucosa from physical and chemical damage. It neutralizes a certain amount of acid and prevents pepsin from coming into contact with the mucosa. On contact with acid, insoluble mucus precipitates into clumps and passes into the duodenum with the chyme. Because mucus is a gel, ions will readily diffuse through it. Therefore it is not the gastric mucosal barrier that prevents the movement of H^+ from the lumen into the cells.

INTRINSIC FACTOR

Intrinsic factor is a mucoprotein with a molecular weight of 55,000 secreted by the parietal cells. It combines with vitamin B_{12} in the stomach, forming a complex that is necessary for the absorption of this vitamin by the ileal mucosa. Failure to secrete intrinsic factor is associated with achlorhydria and the absence of parietal cells, which results in vitamin B_{12} deficiency or pernicious anemia. The development of this disease is poorly understood, for the liver stores enough vitamin B_{12} to last several years. The disease therefore is not recognized until long after the changes have taken place in the gastric mucosa.

GROWTH OF THE MUCOSA

The growth of the gastrointestinal mucosa is influenced by nongastrointestinal hormones and factors associated with the ingestion and digestion of a meal such as gastrointestinal hormones, nervous stimulation, secretions, and trophic substances present in the diet. Hypophysectomy results in atrophy of the digestive tract mucosa and the pancreas. The effects of hypophysectomy on growth can be prevented by administration of growth hormone. When administered to hypophysectomized rats, gastrin prevents atrophy of the gastrointestinal mucosa and exocrine pancreas but does not affect the growth of other tissues. There is interesting evidence that adrenocortical steroids may trigger early postnatal development of the gastrointestinal tract.

Gastrin is an important and necessary regulator of the growth of the oxyntic gland mucosa. It also stimulates growth of the intestinal and colonic mucosa and the exocrine pancreas. In humans antrectomy causes atrophy of the remaining gastric mucosa; in rats it causes atrophy of all gastrointestinal mucosa (except that of the antrum and esophagus) and the exocrine pancreas. These changes are prevented by administration of exogenous gastrin.

Partial resection of the small intestine for tumor removal or for a variety of other reasons (such as treatment of morbid obesity) results in adaptation of the remaining mucosa. The mucosa of the entire digestive tract undergoes hyperplasia, which increases its ability to digest and transport nutrients or, in the case of the stomach, to secrete acid. Resection increases gastrin levels but not sufficiently to account for the adaptive changes. There is evidence that increased exposure of the mucosa to luminal contents plays an important role. After removal of proximal intestine the distal intact mucosa is exposed to an increased load of pancreatic juice, bile, and nutrients. Investigators have hypothesized that bile and pancreatic juice contain growth factors that stimulate the adaptive response. The growth factors have not been isolated and tested. Increased uptake of nutrients by the distal mucosa also has been hypothesized to result in growth. Effects of specific nutrients have not been proved, and there is disagreement whether growth is caused by an increased work load or the increase in the available supply of calories. Good evidence exists that a hormone different from gastrin also is involved in the adaptive response.

The diet also contains polyamines that are required for growth. Trophic agents like gastrin stimulate polyamine synthesis in the proliferative cells. Thus increased luminal polyamines from the diet coupled with synthesis stimulated by trophic hormones may explain the regulation of mucosal growth triggered by changes in the diet.

PATHOPHYSIOLOGY

Gastric and duodenal ulcers are lumped together under the heading of peptic ulcer disease. Although formation of both types of ulcer requires acid and pepsin, their etiologies are basically different. Quite simply, an ulcer forms when damage by acid and pepsin overcomes the ability of the mucosa to protect itself and replace damaged cells. In the case of gastric ulcer the defect more often is in the ability of the mucosa to withstand injury. In

Table 8-1 Comparison of acid output values from the human stomach*

Condition	Representative ranges	
	Basal acid output (mEq/hr)	Maximal acid output (mEq/hr)
Normal	1 to 5	6 to 40
Gastric ulcer	0 to 3	1 to 20
Pernicious anemia	0	0 to 10
Duodenal ulcer	2 to 10	15 to 60
Zollinger-Ellison syndrome (gastrinoma)	10 to 30	30 to 80

*Basal acid output occurs at rest, and maximal acid output during stimulation with histamine. The value is determined by multiplying the hourly volume of gastric juice aspirated times the hydrogen ion concentration of the juice.

the case of duodenal ulcer there is good evidence that the mucosa is exposed to increased amounts of acid and pepsin. This analysis is an oversimplification, for both factors no doubt are important in all cases of ulcer.

Representative acid secretory rates for normal individuals and patients with gastrointestinal disorders are shown in Table 8-1. Maximal acid secretory output sometimes is measured but, in itself, is of little value in diagnosing ulcer disease. Normal subjects secrete approximately 25 mEq H^+/hour, in response to maximal injection of histamine, betazole, or gastrin. The mean output of patients with duodenal ulcer disease is approximately 40 mEq H^+/hour, but the degree of overlap between individuals is so great as to render the determination useless in diagnosis. The highest rates of acid secretion are seen in cases of gastrinoma (Zollinger-Ellison syndrome), but again individual overlap makes it impossible to differentiate between this condition and duodenal ulcer on the basis of secretory data alone. Lower than normal secretory rates are found in cases of gastric ulcer, and still lower secretory rates are found in patients with gastric carcinoma. Many patients in the latter two groups, however, fall well within the normal range.

Because of the feedback mechanism whereby antral acidification inhibits gastrin release, the general statement can be made that serum gastrin levels are related inversely to acid secretory capacity. Patients with gastric ulcer and carcinoma usually have higher than normal serum gastrin levels. Serum gastrin levels in pernicious anemia actually may approach those seen in gastrinoma. Obviously, gastrinoma patients are an exception to this rule because their hypergastrinemia is derived not from the antrum but from a tumor not subject to inhibition by gastric acid. Except for the special tests mentioned in Chapter 1, serum gastrin levels cannot be used to differentiate various secretory abnormalities.

The decreased rate of acid secretion in gastric ulcer is caused in part by the failure to recover acid that has been secreted and then has leaked back across the damaged gastric mucosa. The concept of the gastric mucosal barrier is illustrated in Fig. 8-13. The normal gastric mucosa is relatively impermeable to H^+. If the gastric mucosal barrier is weakened or damaged, H^+ leaks into the mucosa in exchange for Na^+. As H^+ accumulates in the mucosa, intracellular buffers are saturated and pH of the cells decreases, resulting in injury and cell death. Potassium leaks from the dam-

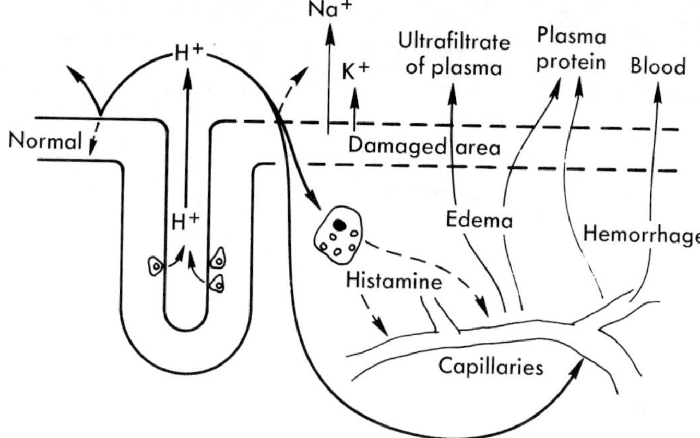

Fig. 8-13. Events that follow damage to the gastric mucosal barrier.

aged cells into the lumen. Hydrogen ion damages mucosal mast cells. They then release histamine, which exacerbates the condition by acting on the mucosal capillaries. The result is local ischemia, hypoxia, and vascular stasis. Plasma proteins and pepsin leak into the gastric juice; and if damage is severe, bleeding occurs. Common agents that produce mucosal damage of this type are aspirin, ethanol, and bile salts. The mucosal lesions produced by topical damage to the gastric barrier may be forerunners of gastric ulcer.

The exact nature of the barrier is unknown. It is probably physiological as well as anatomical. Cell membranes and junctional complexes prevent normal back-diffusion of H^+. Diffused H^+ normally is transported actively back into the lumen. Factors that have been speculated to play a role in maintaining mucosal resistance are blood flow, mucus, cellular renewal, and chemical factors such as gastrin, prostaglandins, and epidermal growth factor. The last three agents have all been shown to decrease the severity and promote the healing of gastric ulcers.

The only factors that have been elucidated as important in duodenal ulcer formation pertain to acid and pepsin secretion. Duodenal ulcer patients have on the average 2 billion parietal cells and can secrete about 40 mEq H^+/hour. Comparable measurements for normal individuals are about 50% of this. In addition the secretion of pepsin is doubled in the duodenal ulcer group, as can be detected by measuring plasma pepsinogen. Although fasting serum gastrin is normal in patients with duodenal ulcer, the gastrin response to a meal and the sensitivity to gastrin are increased. Increased serum gastrin after a meal is caused in part by the fact that acid suppresses gastrin release less effectively in duodenal ulcer patients than in controls. The increased parietal cell mass may therefore be caused by the trophic effect of gastrin.

Medical treatment of duodenal ulcer disease usually consists of administering antacids to neutralize secreted acid or a histamine H_2-receptor blocker to inhibit secretion. A new drug, omeprazole, inhibits the H^+-K^+-ATPase (H^+-pump) directly and blocks all acid secretion. It is extremely effective in treating duodenal ulcers—even those caused by gastrinoma. Surgical treatment is based entirely on physiology. The most commonly employed operations are vagotomy and/or antrectomy. These procedures result in a 60% to 70% decrease in acid secretion by removing one or both major stimulants of acid secretion and their potentiating interaction.

SUGGESTED REFERENCES

Beaumont W: Experiments and observations on the gastric juice and the physiology of digestion, New York, 1955, Dover Publishers, Inc.

Debas HT: Peripheral regulation of gastric acid secretion. In Johnson LR, editor: Physiology of the gastrointestinal tract, ed 2, New York, 1987, Raven Press.

Feldman M and Richardson CT: Gastric acid secretion in humans. In Johnson LR, editor: Physiology of the gastrointestinal tract, New York, 1981, Raven Press.

Forte JG and Wolosin JM: HCl secretion by the gastric oxyntic cell. In Johnson LR, editor: Physiology of the gastrointestinal tract, ed 2, New York, 1987, Raven Press.

Hersey SJ: Pepsinogen secretion. In Johnson LR, editor: Physiology of the gastrointestinal tract, ed 2, New York, 1987, Raven Press.

Johnson LR: Regulation of gastrointestinal growth. In Johnson LR, editor: Physiology of the gastrointestinal tract, ed 2, New York, 1987, Raven Press.

Robert A, Nezamis JE, Lancaster C, and Hanchar AJ: Cytoprotection by prostaglandins in rats. Prevention of gastric necrosis produced by alcohol, HCl, NaOH, hypertonic NaCl, and thermal injury, Gastroenterology 77:433-443, 1979.

Sachs G: The gastric proton pump: the H^+-K^+ ATPase. In Johnson LR, editor: Physiology of the gastrointestinal tract, ed 2, New York, 1987, Raven Press.

Saffouri B, DuVal JW, and Makhlouf GM: Stimulation of gastrin secretion *in vitro* by intraluminal chemicals: regulation by intramural cholinergic and noncholinergic neurons, Gastroenterology 87:557-561, 1984.

Silen W: Gastric mucosal defense and repair. In Johnson LR, editor: Physiology of the gastrointestinal tract, ed 2, New York, 1987, Raven Press.

Soll AH: Physiology of isolated gastric glands and parietal cells: receptors and effectors regulating function. In Johnson LR: Physiology of the gastrointestinal tract, ed 2, New York, 1987, Raven Press.

9 Pancreatic Secretion

Leonard R. Johnson

Pancreatic exocrine secretion is divided conveniently into an aqueous or bicarbonate component and an enzymatic component. The function of the aqueous component is the neutralization of the duodenal contents. As such it prevents damage to the duodenal mucosa by acid and pepsin and brings the pH of the contents into the optimum range for activity of the pancreatic enzymes. The enzymatic or protein component is a low-volume secretion containing enzymes for the digestion of all normal constituents of a meal. Unlike the enzymes secreted by the stomach and salivary glands the pancreatic enzymes are essential to normal digestion and absorption.

FUNCTIONAL ANATOMY

The exocrine pancreas can best be likened to a cluster of grapes, and its functional units resemble the salivons of the salivary glands. Groups of acini form lobules separated by areolar tissue. Each acinus is formed from several pyramidal acinar cells oriented with their apices toward the lumen. The lumen of the spherical acinus is drained by a ductule whose epithelium extends into the acinus in the form of centroacinar cells. Ductules join to form intralobular ducts, which in turn drain into interlobular ducts. These join the major pancreatic duct draining the gland.

The acinar cells secrete a small volume of juice rich in protein. Essentially all the proteins present in pancreatic juice are digestive enzymes. Ductule cells and centroacinar cells produce a large volume of watery secretion containing Na^+ and HCO_3^- as its major constituents.

Distributed throughout the pancreatic parenchyma are the islets of Langerhans or the endocrine pancreas. The islets produce insulin from the β cells and glucagon from the α cells. In addition, the pancreas produces the candidate hormone, pancreatic polypeptide, and contains large amounts of somatostatin, which may act as a paracrine to inhibit the release of insulin and glucagon.

The efferent nerve supply to the pancreas includes both sympathetics and parasympathetics. Sympathetic postganglionic fibers emanate from the celiac and superior mesenteric

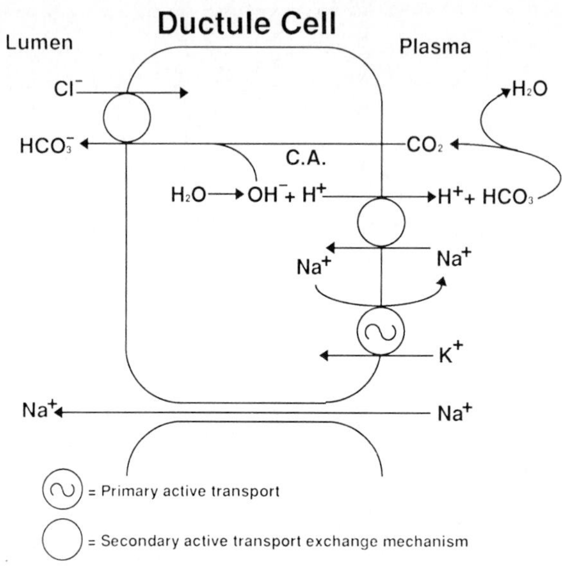

Fig. 9-1. The biochemical and transport processes necessary for secretion of the aqueous component of pancreatic juice.

plexuses and accompany the arteries to the organ. Parasympathetic preganglionic fibers are distributed by branches of the vagi coursing down the antral-duodenal region. Hence, surgical vagotomy for peptic ulcer disease affects not only the intended target organ, the hypersecreting stomach, but also the pancreas. Recently more selective operations have been designed to resect only the vagal branches passing to the stomach. Vagal fibers terminate at either acini and islets or intrinsic cholinergic nerves of the pancreas. In general the sympathetic nerves inhibit and the parasympathetic nerves stimulate pancreatic exocrine secretion.

MECHANISMS OF FLUID AND ELECTROLYTE SECRETION

The pancreas secretes approximately 1 L of fluid per day. At all rates of secretion, pancreatic juice is essentially isotonic with extracellular fluid. At low rates the primary ions are Na^+ and Cl^-. At high rates Na^+ and HCO_3^- predominate. Potassium ions are present at all rates of secretion at a concentration equal to their concentration in plasma. The concentrations of Na^+ in pancreatic juice and plasma are also approximately equal.

The aqueous component is secreted by the ductule and centroacinar cells and may contain 120 to 140 mEq HCO_3^-/L, several times its concentration in plasma. The electropotential difference across the ductule epithelium is 5 to 9 mV, lumen negative. Hence HCO_3^- is secreted against both electrical and chemical gradients. This is often considered evidence that HCO_3^- is transported actively across the luminal surface of the cells. Recent evidence, however, suggests that secretion of HCO_3^- depends on the Na^+ gradient established by the Na^+-K^+-ATPase in the basolateral membrane (Fig. 9-1). This creates an electrochemical gradient for Na^+ to diffuse into the cell. It exchanges for H^+ moving out of the cell against its gradient. This in turn allows CO_2 to move readily into the alkalinized cell, combining with OH^- to form HCO_3^-. The combination of CO_2 with water is catalyzed by carbonic an-

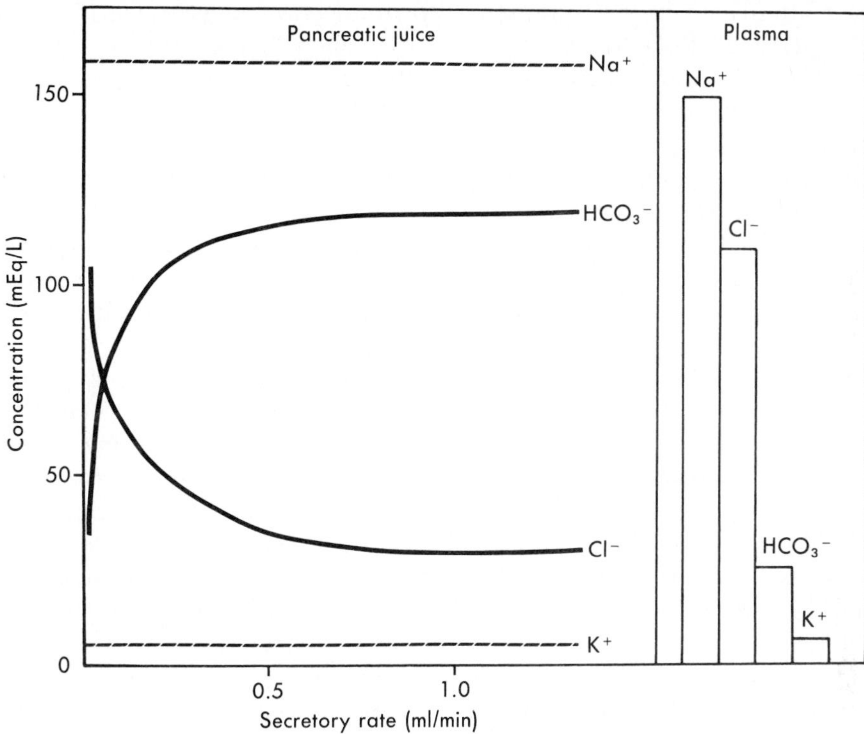

Fig. 9-2. Relationship between the rate of secretion of pancreatic juice and the concentrations of its major ions.

hydrase. As H^+ continues to leave the cell, HCO_3^- accumulates within and moves across the apical membrane in exchange for Cl^-. When H^+ reaches the plasma it combines with HCO_3^- to produce additional CO_2 that may diffuse into the cell. Na^+ moves down the established electrochemical gradient from the plasma to the lumen of the gland. Water passively moves from the plasma across the cells into the lumen, down the osmotic gradient created by the secretion of Na^+ and HCO_3^-. This secretion is similar to that occurring in the parietal cells of the stomach, except that the H^+ and HCO_3^- are transported in opposite directions. Thus the venous blood from an actively secreting pancreas has a lower pH than that from an inactive gland.

As in gastric juice the ionic concentrations in pancreatic juice vary with the rates of secretion (Fig. 9-2). The concentrations of anions (Cl^- and HCO_3^-) in pancreatic juice are related inversely to each other, as are the concentrations of cations (Na^+ and H^+) in gastric juice. Because these relationships are analogous it might be surmised that analogous theories have been proposed to explain them.

- The two-component hypothesis assumes that one cell type, perhaps the acinar cell, secretes a small amount of fluid whose major ions are Na^+ and Cl^-. Other cell types, the ductule and centroacinar cells, secrete large volumes of juice rich in Na^+ and HCO_3^- in response to stimulation. At low rates of secretion the Cl^- concentration of the juice is therefore relatively high. As the secretory rate increases the fixed amount of Cl^- being secreted is diluted by the much larger volume of HCO_3^--containing juice and the final concentrations of the two anions approach the pure HCO_3^- secretion.

- Another theory proposes that the cells primarily secrete HCO_3^- and that, as it moves down the ducts, it is exchanged for Cl^-. At low rates of secretion there is sufficient time for exchange to be nearly complete, and the concentration of each anion is equal to its concentration in plasma. As the rate of secretion increases, less time is available for exchange, and the final ionic makeup of pancreatic juice approaches that of the originally secreted solution containing only HCO_3^- and Na^+. Both processes are probably involved in determining the final makeup of the secreted juice.

MECHANISMS OF ENZYME SECRETION

The pancreatic acinar cells synthesize and secrete major enzymes for the digestion of all three primary foodstuffs. Like pepsin, the pancreatic proteases are secreted as inactive enzyme precursors and are converted to active forms in the lumen. Pancreatic amylase and lipase are secreted in active forms. The activation and specific actions of the pancreatic enzymes are covered in detail in Chapter 11.

Although a certain amount of controversy exists concerning the mechanisms involved in the synthesis and secretion of enzymes by the acinar cells, the process outlined in Fig. 9-3 is accepted by most authorities. The secretory process begins with the synthesis of exportable proteins in association with polysomes attached to the cisternae of the rough endoplasmic reticulum (step *1*). As it is being synthesized the elongating protein enters the cisternal cavity, where it is collected after synthesis has become complete (step *2*). Once within the cisternal space, enzymes remain membrane-bound until they are secreted from the cell. They next move through the cisternae of the rough endoplasmic reticulum to transitional elements, which are associated with smooth vesicles at the Golgi periphery. Possibly as a result of pinching off the transitional elements containing them, the enzymes become associated with the Golgi vesicles (step *3*), which transport them to condensing vacuoles (step *4*), Energy is required for the transport through the endoplasmic reticulum and Golgi vesicles to the condensing vacuoles. Within the condensing vacuoles the enzymes are concentrated to form zymogen granules (step *5*). They then are stored in the zymogen granules that collect at the apex of the cell. After a secretory stimulus the membrane of the zymogen granule fuses with the cell membrane, ultimately rupturing and expelling the enzymes into the lumen (step *6*). This is the only step in the process that requires a secretory stimulus.

REGULATION OF SECRETION

As might be expected from its function to neutralize the duodenum, the secretion of fluid and HCO_3^- (the aqueous component) largely is determined by the amount of acid entering the duodenum. The secretion of pancreatic enzymes is, similarly, determined primarily by the amount of fat and protein entering the duodenum. Control of pancreatic secretion is regulated primarily by secretin, cholecystokinin, and vagovagal reflexes. Intestinal stimuli account for most pancreatic secretion, but secretion also is stimulated during the cephalic and gastric phases.

Basal pancreatic secretion in humans is low and difficult to measure. The basal secretion of bicarbonate is 2% to 3% of maximal, and basal enzyme secretion is 10% to 15% of maximal. The stimuli for basal secretion are unknown.

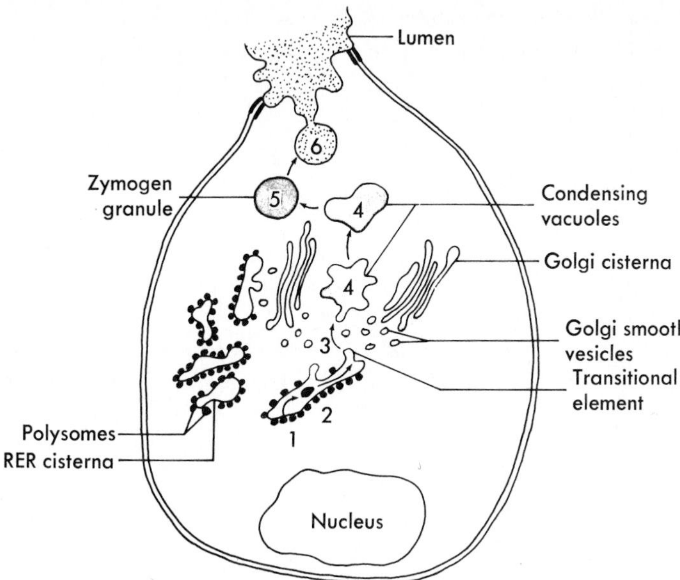

Fig. 9-3. Pancreatic acinar cell. Note the major steps in the cellular synthesis and secretion of enzymes. See text for an explanation of steps *1* through *6*.

Because the isolated perfused pancreas secretes basally, this secretion may be an intrinsic property of the gland.

Cephalic Phase

Truncal vagotomy reduces the pancreatic secretory response to a meal by approximately 60%. Most of this decrease is caused by the interruption of vagovagal reflexes and by the removal of the potentiating and sensitizing effects of acetylcholine, which increase the response to secretin.

There is, however, a direct vagal component of stimulation that is initiated during the cephalic phase. Sham-feeding produces a pancreatic secretory response, which, of course, is blocked totally by vagotomy. In dogs the cephalic phase accounts for approximately 20% of the response to a meal. The stimuli for the cephalic phase of pancreatic secretion are the conditioned reflexes, smell, taste, chewing, and swallowing. Afferent impulses travel to the vagal nucleus. Vagal efferents to the pancreas stimulate both the ductule and the acinar cells to secrete. Stimulation is mediated by acetylcholine and has a greater effect on the enzymatic component than it does on the aqueous component. In dogs a portion of the cephalic phase is mediated by gastrin released by the vagus. Gastrin has about half the potency of cholecystokinin for activating the acinar cells. Gastrin plays only a minor role in the regulation of human pancreatic secretion. These mechanisms are illustrated in Fig. 9-4.

Gastric Phase

The stimulation of pancreatic secretion originating from food in the stomach is mediated by the same mechanisms that are involved in the cephalic phase. Distention of the wall of the stomach initiates vagovagal reflexes to the pancreas. Gastrin is released by protein digestion products and distention. (See Chapter 8.)

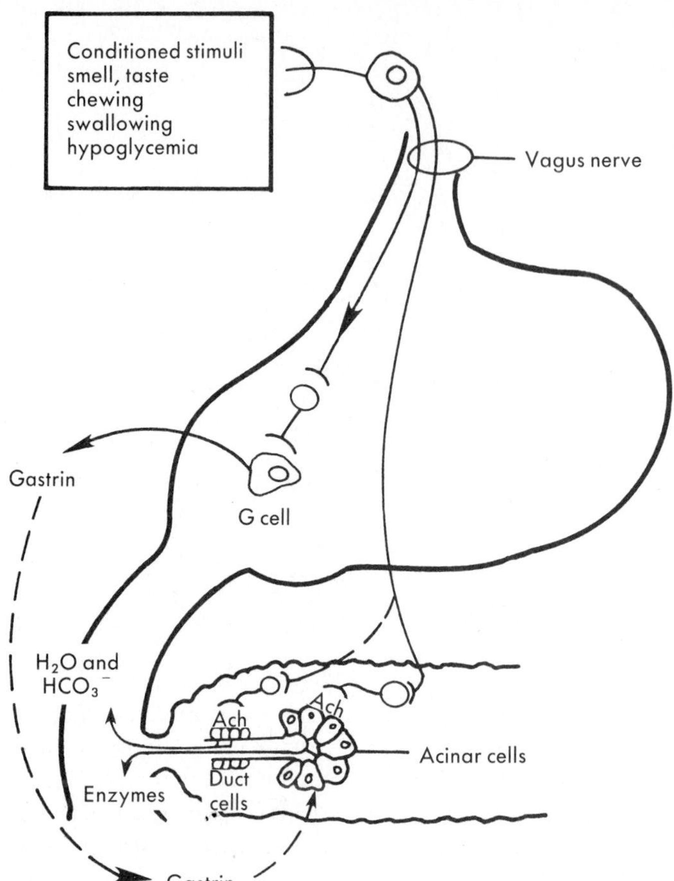

Fig. 9-4. Mechanisms involved in the stimulation of pancreatic secretion during the cephalic phase. *Dashed lines* represent minor effects.

Intestinal Phase

The presence of digestion products and hydrogen ions in the human small intestine accounts for 70% to 80% of the stimulation of pancreatic secretion. Secretin and cholecystokinin account for almost all the hormonal stimulation of pancreatic secretion. The stimulus for the alkaline component (water and bicarbonate) is secretin released from the S cells by gastric acid and high concentrations of long-chain fatty acids. Secretion of the enzymatic component from the acinar cells is stimulated by CCK released from the I cells by fat and protein digestion products. Cholinergic reflexes also stimulate the acinar cells because vagotomy markedly reduces the enzymatic response.

The only potent releaser of secretin is hydrogen ion. The duodenal pH threshold for secretin release is 4.5. Secretin release rises almost linearly as the pH is lowered to 3 (Fig. 9-5). Lowering the pH below 3 does not lead to greater release of secretin, provided the amount of titratable acid entering the duodenum is held constant. Below pH 3, secretin release and pancreatic bicarbonate secretion are

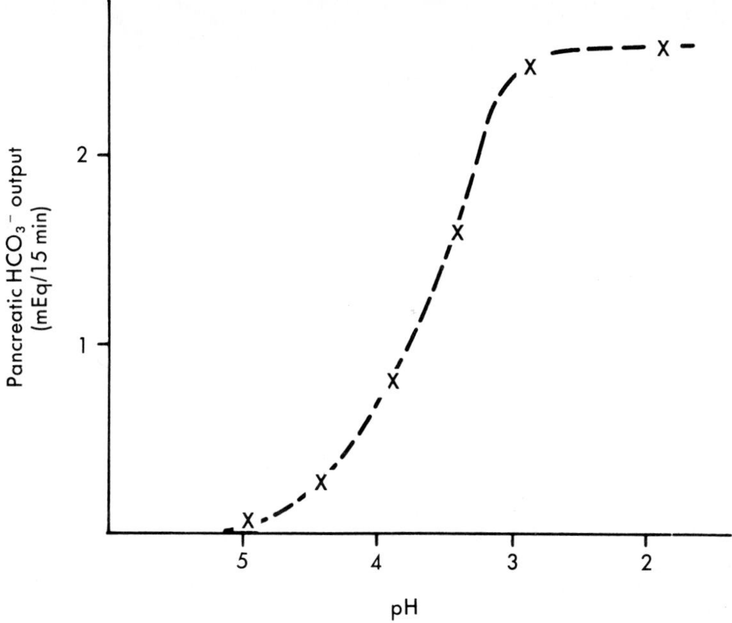

Fig. 9-5. Pancreatic bicarbonate output in response to various duodenal pH values. The output of bicarbonate is used as an index of secretin release.

related only to the amount of titratable acid entering the duodenum per unit of time. As more acid enters the gut, more secretin-containing cells are stimulated to release hormone. Thus at a constant pH the amount of secretin released is a function of the length of gut acidified. Secretin can be released from the entire duodenum and jejunum, and the amount of hormone available for release appears to be constant per centimeter of proximal small intestine.

During the response to a normal meal, however, only the duodenal bulb and proximal duodenum are acidified sufficiently to release secretin. The pH of the proximal duodenum rarely drops below 4 to 3.5. This raises doubts concerning whether sufficient secretin is released by a meal to account for the high rates of pancreatic bicarbonate and water secretion normally seen. If the pH of the gastric contents entering the duodenum is kept at 5 or higher by automatic titration, the pancreatic response is typical of CCK and acetylcholine acting alone (a small volume of enzyme-rich juice). Dropping the pH even slightly below the threshold for secretin release leads to large increases in volume and bicarbonate secretion. The conclusion therefore is that the effects of a small amount of secretin are potentiated by CCK and acetylcholine.

This is an important physiological interaction of two gastrointestinal hormones and cholinergic reflexes and is demonstrated directly by the experiment outlined in Fig. 9-6. Phenylalanine, a potent releaser of CCK and initiator of vagovagal reflexes, produces a small increase in volume when given alone. If, however, the same dose is infused into the gut while a low dose of secretin is given intravenously, the output of the pancreatic alkaline component increases to levels seen during a meal. Vagotomy greatly decreases the

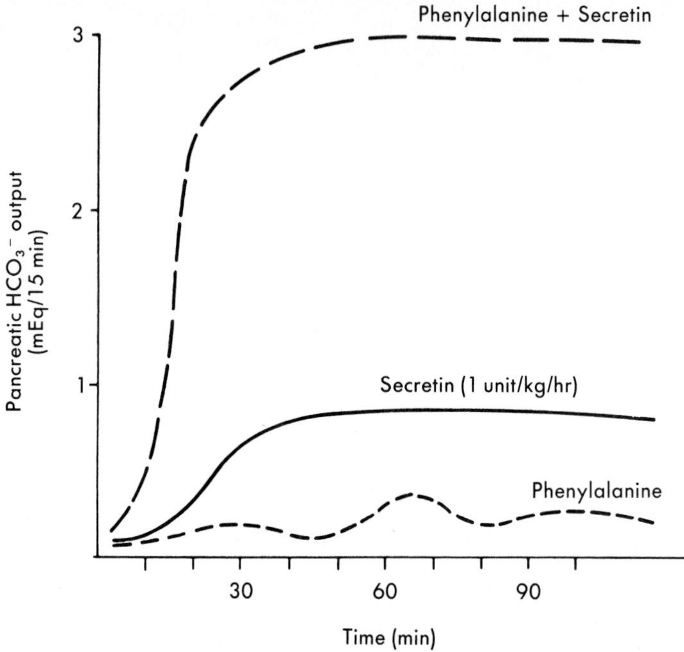

Fig. 9-6. Pancreatic bicarbonate output in response to continual perfusion of the duodenum with phenylalanine, to continuous intravenous infusion of secretin, and to the combination of the two stimuli. Note that the response to secretin is greatly potentiated by endogenous phenylalanine.

potentiated response. Physiologically, then, the volume and bicarbonate response to a meal result from acetylcholine and CCK, which potentiate the effect of the small amount of secretin released by duodenal acidification.

Secretin has been referred to as "nature's antacid" because most of its physiological and pharmacological actions decrease the amount of acid in the duodenum. For example, it stimulates secretion of HCO_3^- from the pancreas and liver and inhibits gastric secretion and emptying as well as gastrin release.

CCK is the principal humoral stimulant of enzyme secretion from the pancreatic acinar cells. It is released in response to amino acids and fatty acids in the small intestine. Only L-isomers of amino acids are effective. In dogs, phenylalanine and tryptophan are potent releasers. Alanine, leucine, and valine are less effective. Phenylalanine, methionine, and valine appear to be potent releasers in humans. CCK is distributed evenly over the first 90 cm of intestine, and infusion of L-phenylalanine below the ligament of Treitz produces pancreatic enzyme responses equal to those seen after infusion near the pylorus. Thus the amount of CCK released depends on the load and length of bowel exposed as well as on the concentration of amino acids present.

There is strong evidence that some peptides as well as single amino acids also release CCK. Three dipeptides, all of which contain glycine (glycylphenylalanine, glycyltryptophan, phenylalanylglycine), are effective. Dipeptides or tripeptides of glycine, or glycine it-

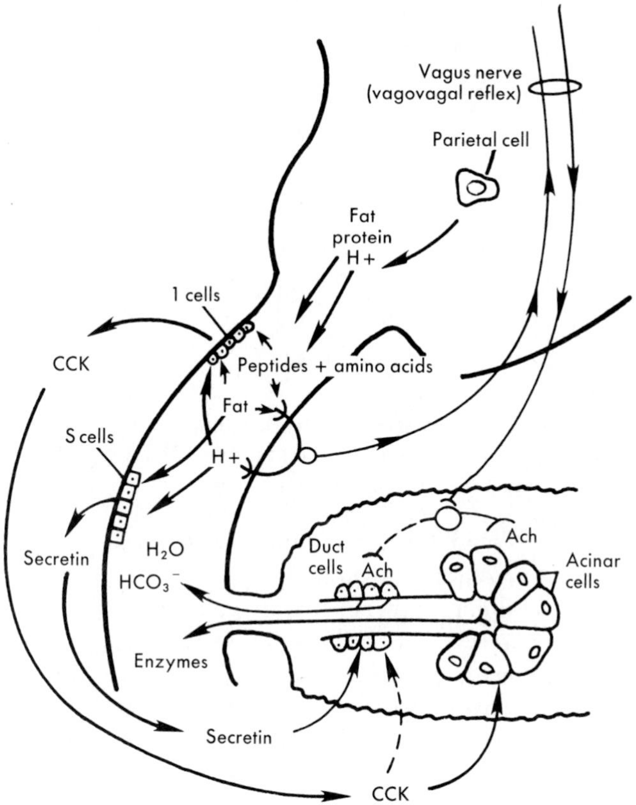

Fig. 9-7. Mechanisms involved in the stimulation of pancreatic secretion during the intestinal phase. *Dashed lines* indicate potentiative interactions with secretin.

self, are ineffective. There is evidence that some peptides containing at least four amino acids are also effective. Undigested protein does not release CCK. After a protein meal, therefore, a wide variety of specific protein products evoke CCK release and pancreatic enzyme secretion.

In addition to protein products, fatty acids longer than eight carbon atoms release CCK and initiate vagovagal reflexes. Lauric, palmitic, stearic, and oleic acids are equal and strong releasers of CCK. Fat must be in an absorbable form before release of the hormone occurs. The interactions between luminal nutrients and the receptors triggering the release of CCK, and of gastrointestinal hormones in general, are poorly understood. As a result, most of the intracellular mechanisms resulting in hormone release are unknown. Part of the reason for this paucity of information has been the inability to isolate large numbers of hormone-containing cells from the mucosa of the gastrointestinal tract.

The mechanisms resulting in the stimulation of pancreatic secretion during the intestinal phase are illustrated in Fig. 9-7.

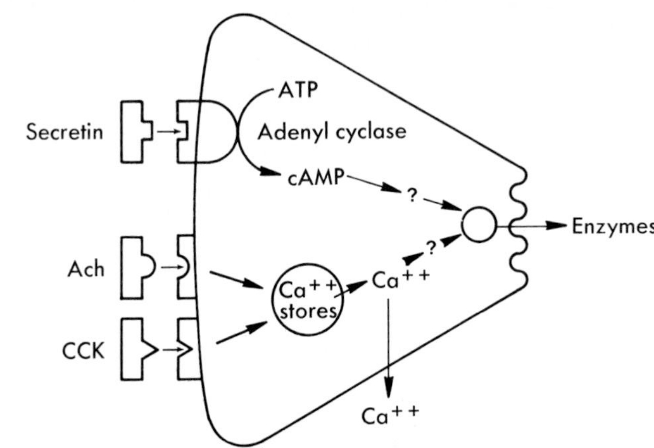

Fig. 9-8. Receptors on the rodent pancreatic acinar cell. Different second messengers for the stimulants indicate different cellular mechanisms for stimulation and provide the basis for potentiation.

CELLULAR BASIS FOR POTENTIATION

The concept of potentiation requires that the potentiating stimuli act on different membrane receptors and trigger different cellular mechanisms for the stimulation of secretion. Some of the steps in these mechanisms have been elucidated for the pancreatic acinar cell and are illustrated in Fig. 9-8. Secretin binding to its receptor triggers an increase in adenylyl cyclase activity, resulting in the synthesis of cyclic AMP. Acetylcholine and CCK bind to separate receptors, but both increase intracellular Ca^{++}. The Ca^{++} is mobilized primarily from the plasma membranes and rough endoplasmic retriculum of the acinar cells. Both CCK and acetylcholine also increase diacylglycerol and inositol trisphosphate production from phosphatidylinositol. It is likely that one of these breakdown products is the intracellular messenger for Ca^{++} release. Interactions between secretin and acetylcholine or secretin and CCK result in potentiation. However, the effects of combining CCK and acetylcholine, which trigger identical mechanisms, are only additive.

The final steps in the process leading to enzyme secretion have not been elucidated, but they involve the phosphorylation of structural and regulatory proteins. Potentiation occurs because Ca^{++} and cAMP phosphorylate different proteins. The foregoing interactions have been worked out with guinea pig isolated pancreatic acini. Secretin does not potentiate the effects of CCK and acetylcholine in dogs or humans. A system similar to this, however, is a likely explanation of the potentiation in all species in which it occurs. Thus similar events may be predicted for the human ductule cell.

RESPONSE TO A MEAL

As digestion and mixing of food proceed in the stomach, buffers present in proteins and peptides become saturated with hydrogen ions and the pH drops to about 2.0. The maximum load of titratable acid (free H^+ plus bound H^+) delivered to the duodenum is 20 to 30 mEq per hour. This is approximately equal to the maximal capacity of the stomach to secrete acid, which, in turn, equals the ability of the pancreas to secrete HCO_3^- when it is maximally stimulated. To raise the pH of the duodenum the undissociated H^+ as well as the free H^+ must be neutralized. This is accomplished rapidly in the first part of the duodenum and the pH of the chyme is raised quickly from 2.0 at the pylorus to above 4.0 beyond the duodenal bulb. Some neutralization occurs by absorption of H^+ and secretion of bicarbonate by the gut wall. An additional amount of H^+ is neutralized by HCO_3^- in the bile. The contributions of the gut mucosa and bile, however, are small, and by far the greatest proportion of acid is neutralized by the large volume of pancreatic juice secreted into the lumen.

Within a few minutes after chyme enters the duodenum there is a sharp rise in the secretion of pancreatic enzymes. Within 30 minutes enzyme secretion peaks at levels about 70% to 80% of those attainable with maximal stimulation by CCK and cholinergic reflexes. Enzyme secretion continues at this rate until the stomach is empty. The enzyme response to a meal may be kept below maximum by the presence of humoral inhibitors of pancreatic secretion. This is the proposed function of pancreatic polypeptide.

CLINICAL APPLICATIONS

Abnormal pancreatic secretion occurs in diseases such as chronic and acute pancreatitis, cystic fibrosis, and kwashiorkor, and in tumors that involve the gland itself. Changes in secretion during one of these diseases depend upon the stage of development of the disease. Most patients with chronic pancreatitis have decreased volume and bicarbonate output, whereas those with acute pancreatitis often have normal secretion. Both volume and enzyme content of pancreatic juice are decreased by cystic fibrosis. Tumors of the pancreas frequently decrease the volume of secretion. In kwashiorkor, both the alkaline and the enzymatic components are depressed, but amylase secretion continues after trypsin, chymotrypsin, and lipase activities are no longer found.

Pancreatic enzyme secretion must be reduced by more than 80% to produce steatorrhea. If a patient has steatorrhea, it is only necessary to measure the concentration of any pancreatic enzyme in the jejunal content after a meal to determine whether the condition is pancreatic in origin.

Pancreatic exocrine function is assessed by measuring basal secretion and secretion stimulated by secretin and/or CCK. These function tests are performed on a fasting patient. A double-lumen nasogastric tube is used. One tube opens into the stomach to drain gastric contents that would otherwise empty into the duodenum; the other collects duodenal juice that is assumed to be largely pancreatic in origin. Interpretation of the test is impeded by contaminating biliary secretions. Changes in secretion depend upon the stage of development of various diseases and may vary from patient to patient. For these reasons, pancreatic function tests are not reliable in the diagnosis of individual diseases but are used to assess overall pancreatic function.

SELECTED REFERENCES

Anagostides A, Chadwick VS, Selden AC, and Maton PN: Sham feeding and pancreatic secretion; evidence for direct vagal stimulation of enzyme output, Gastroenterology 87:109-114, 1984.

Beglinger C, Grossman MI, and Solomon TE: Interaction between stimulants of exocrine pancreatic secretion in dogs, Am J Physiol 246:G173-G179, 1984.

Beglinger C, Taylor IL, Grossman MI, and Solomon TE: Pancreatic polypeptide inhibits exocrine pancreatic secretion to six stimulants, Am J Physiol 246:G286-G291, 1984.

Gardner JD and Jeuseu RT: Secretagogue receptors on pancreatic acinar cells. In Johnson LR, editor: Physiology of the gastrointestinal tract, ed 2, New York, 1987, Raven Press.

Gorelick FS and Jamieson JD: Structure-function relationship of the pancreas. In Johnson LR, editor: Physiology of the gastrointestinal tract, ed 2, New York, 1987, Raven Press.

Hootman SR and Williams JA: Stimulus-secretion coupling in the pancreatic acinus. In Johnson LR, editor: Physiology of the gastrointestinal tract, ed 2, New York, 1987, Raven Press.

Meyer JH, Kelley GA, Spingola LJ, and Jones RS: Canine gut receptors mediating pancreatic responses to luminal L-amino acids, Am J Physiol 231:669-677, 1976.

Meyer JH, Way LW, and Grossman MI: Pancreatic response to acidification of various lengths of proximal intestine in the dog, Am J Physiol 219:971-977, 1970.

Schulz I: Electrolyte and fluid secretion in the exocrine pancreas. In Johnson LR, editor: Physiology of the gastrointestinal tract, ed 2, New York, 1987, Raven Press.

Solomon TE: Control of exocrine pancreatic secretion. In Johnson LR, editor: Physiology of the gastrointestinal tract, ed 2, New York, 1987, Raven Press.

Solomon TE, and Grossman MI: Effect of atropine and vagotomy on response of transplanted pancreas, Am J Physiol 236:E186-E190, 1979.

10 Bile Production, Secretion, and Storage

Norman W. Weisbrodt

Secretion of bile is necessary for the proper digestion and absorption of lipids. It also is required for the normal elimination of various endogenous products (e.g., cholesterol and bile pigments) as well as exogenously administered chemicals (e.g., phenothiazines and heavy metals). Bile secretion here will be discussed in three parts: (1) the formation of bile by the hepatocytes and biliary ducts; (2) the storage and concentration of bile in the gallbladder; and (3) the expulsion and transport of bile from the gallbladder to the lumen of the intestine.

BILE FORMATION

Constituents of Bile

Bile is a complex mixture of organic and inorganic components. Taken separately, some of the components are insoluble and would precipitate out of an aqueous medium. Normally, however, bile is a homogeneous and stable solution whose stability depends upon the physical behavior and interactions of its various components.

Bile acids are the major organic constituents of bile, accounting for approximately 50% of the solid components. Chemically they are carboxylic acids with a cyclopentanophenanthrene nucleus and a branched side chain of three to nine carbon atoms that ends in a carboxyl group (Fig. 10-1). They are related structurally to cholesterol, from which they are synthesized by the liver. Several features are unique to the bile acids and account for their behavior in solution. Three dimensionally the hydroxyl and carboxyl groups are located on one side of the molecule. The bulk of the molecule is composed of the nucleus and several methyl groups (Fig. 10-1). This structure renders bile acids amphipathic, to the extent that the hydroxyl and dissociated carboxyl groups are hydrophilic and the nucleus and methyl groupings are hydrophobic. In solution the behavior of bile acids depends on their concentration. At low concentrations there is little interaction between bile acid molecules. As the concentration is increased a point is reached where aggregation of the molecules takes place. These aggregates are called "micelles," and the point of formation

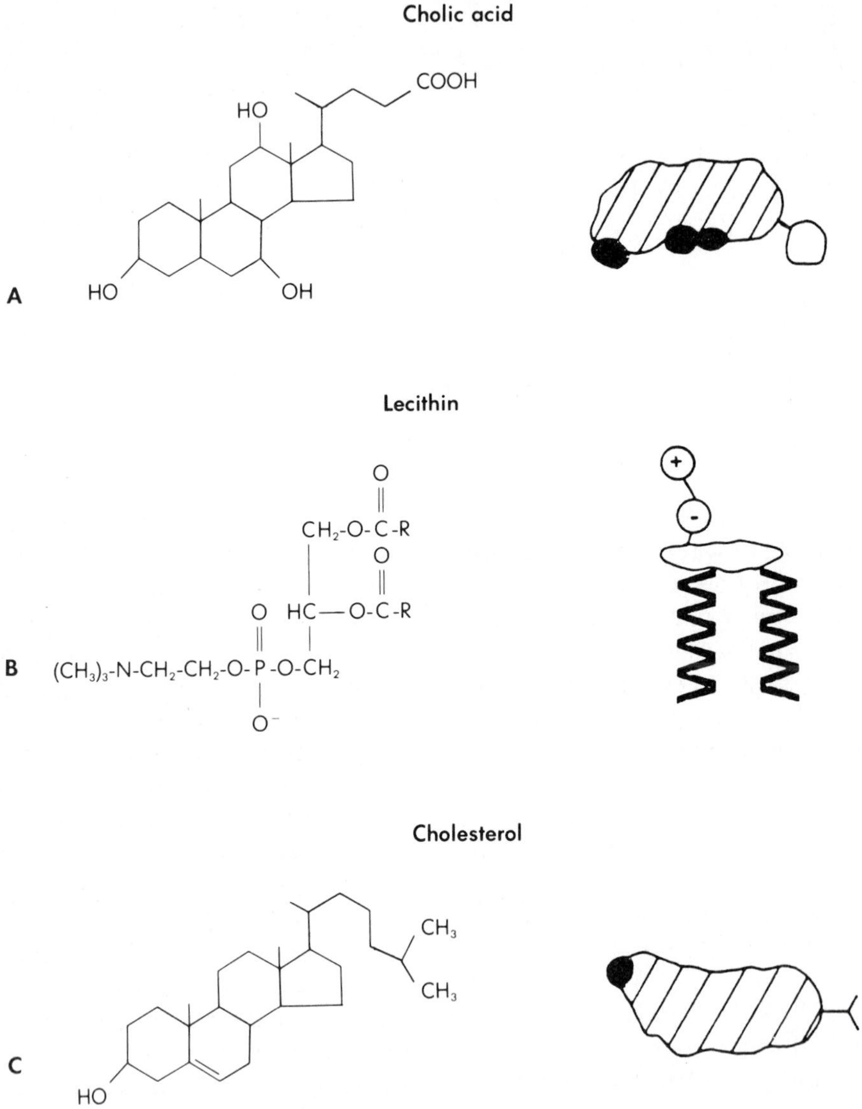

Cholic acid

COOH

HO

A HO OH

Lecithin

O

||

CH_2-O-C-R

O

||

O HC—O-C-R

||

B $(CH_3)_3$-N-CH_2-CH_2-O-P-O-CH_2

O^-

Cholesterol

CH_3

CH_3

C

HO

Fig. 10-1. Structural formulas for some of the components of bile. *Left,* Conventional representation; *right,* shorthand version of the Stuart-Briegleb representation. **A**, Cholic acid. Note that the polar hydroxyl groups *(dark circles)* and the carboxyl group are on the same side of the molecule. **B**, Lecithin. Note that the polar phosphatidylcholine group is at one end and the nonpolar fatty acids are at the other. **C**, Cholesterol. Only one hydroxyl group is present; thus cholesterol is strongly hydrophobic.

is called the "critical micellar concentration." Hydrophobic regions of the micelles interact with one another, and the hydrophilic regions interact with the water molecules (see Fig. 11-13).

The most common human bile acids are cholic acid, chenodeoxycholic acid, deoxycholic acid, and lithocholic acid. These differ from one another primarily in the number of hydroxyl groups present. Cholic acid is a trihydroxy acid; deoxycholic acid and chenodeoxycholic acid are dihydroxy acids; lithocholic acid is a monohydroxy acid and is only slightly soluble. Another feature that affects the aqueous solubility of bile acids is the state of the terminal carboxyl group. The pK of bile acids is almost neutral; thus at the pH of duodenal contents the acids are undissociated and relatively insoluble. Most bile acids, however, exist not as free acids but as conjugates of taurine or glycine. Conjugated bile salts therefore have much lower pK values and exist as the more soluble dissociated salts at pH values that are found in the biliary tract and duodenum.

The second most abundant group of organic compounds in bile are the phospholipids, the major ones being the lecithins (Fig. 10-1). Phospholipids are also amphipathic, insofar as the phosphatidylcholine grouping is hydrophilic, whereas the fatty acid chains are hydrophobic. Although amphipathic the phospholipids are not soluble in water but form liquid crystals that swell in solution. In the presence of bile salts, however, the liquid crystals are broken up and solubilized as a component of the micelles. Bile salts possess a large capacity to solubilize phospholipids; 2 mol of lecithin are solubilized by 1 mol of bile salts. The combination of bile salts and phospholipids is also better able to solubilize other lipids—mainly cholesterol—than is a simple solution of bile salts.

A third organic component, cholesterol, is present in small amounts, contributing about 4% to the total solids of bile. Although present in small amounts, bile cholesterol is important because it may be excreted to help regulate body stores of cholesterol. Cholesterol appears mainly in the nonesterified form and is insoluble in water. In the presence of bile salts and phospholipids, however, it is solubilized as part of the micelle. Because it is a weakly polar substance, cholesterol is found in the interior of the micelle, where the hydrophobic portions of the bile salts and phospholipids interact.

The fourth major group of organic compounds found in bile are the bile pigments. These constitute only 2% of the total solids, with bilirubin being the most important. Chemically, bile pigments are tetrapyrroles and are related to the porphyrins, from which they are derived. In their free form, bile pigments are insoluble in water. Normally, however, they are conjugated with glucuronic acid and rendered soluble. Unlike the other organic compounds just mentioned, bile pigments do not take part in micellar formation. As their name implies they are highly colored substances. Other than being responsible for the normal color of bile and feces, the pigment properties of these compounds are utilized to assess the level of function of the liver (see pp. 106–107).

In addition to the organic compounds just discussed, many inorganic ions are found in bile. The predominant cation is Na^+, accompanied by smaller amounts of K^+ and Ca^{++}. The predominant inorganic anions are Cl^- and HCO_3^-. Normally the total number of inorganic cations will exceed the total number of inorganic anions. There is no anion deficit, however, because the bile acids, which possess a net negative charge at the pH values found in bile, account for the difference. Because they are highly charged molecules the bile acids attract a layer of cations that serve

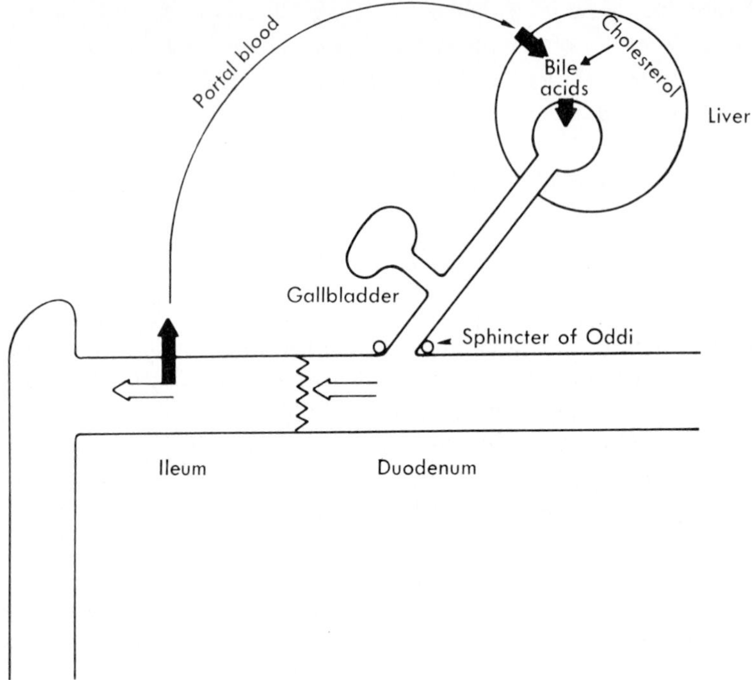

Fig. 10-2. Enterohepatic circulation of bile acids. These acids are actively secreted by the liver. Once in the intestine they participate in the digestion and absorption of lipids. As they are propelled toward the distal small bowel, some of the "primary" acids are altered, becoming "secondary" acids. These, along with the "primary" ones, are absorbed actively from the terminal ileum. However, a minor fraction of both types is not absorbed but is propelled into the colon. The absorbed bile acids are transported via the portal circulation to the liver, where they are extracted actively from the blood (almost 100%) and resecreted. Synthesis of new "primary" acids from cholesterol occurs at a rate to compensate for the acids lost from the bowel. *Solid arrows* denote active absorption, secretion, and synthesis; *open arrows,* propulsion of contents by contractions of the intestine.

as counterions. These counterions are tightly associated with the micelles and exert little osmotic activity. Thus bile is isosmotic even though there is a larger number of cations present than expected.

SECRETION OF BILE

The secretion of bile depends heavily upon the secretion of bile acids by the liver. Once secreted, bile acids undergo an interesting journey (Fig. 10-2). First, they may be stored in the gallbladder. Then they are propelled into and through the small intestine, where they take part in the digestion and absorption of lipids. In the terminal ileum, most of the bile acids are absorbed actively and travel in the portal blood to the liver. In the liver they are taken up by the hepatocytes and resecreted. This process is termed the "enterohepatic circulation."

Bile acids are secreted continuously by the liver. The rate of secretion, however, varies widely. Early experiments demonstrated that the rate of secretion depended on the amount of bile acid delivered to the liver in the blood; the more acid in the portal blood, the greater the secretion of bile. The amount of bile acid in the portal blood depends upon the amount absorbed from the small intestine. The amount of bile acid in the intestine, in turn, depends upon the digestive state of the individual. Between meals, most bile secreted by the liver is stored in the gallbladder (pp. 105–106) rather than delivered to the small intestine. During a meal the gallbladder empties its contents into the duodenum. Bile acids are then resorbed in the terminal ileum by a highly efficient active transport process, and the cycle continues. It is estimated that the total amount of bile acid in the body is secreted twice during the digestion of each meal.

The enterohepatic circulation of bile acids is characterized by the active transport of the acids at two locations, the ileum and the hepatocytes. The hepatocytes actively remove bile acid from the blood by a process that is normally efficient: practically all bile acids are removed during one passage through the liver. The process does have a transport maximum, but this is seldom reached.

Cholic and chenodeoxycholic acids are called primary bile acids, meaning that they are synthesized by human hepatocytes. Their synthesis by the liver is a continuous but regulated process. The amount synthesized depends upon the amount of bile acid returned to the liver in the enterohepatic circulation. If most of the bile acids secreted by the liver are returned, synthesis is low; but if the secreted acids are lost from the enterohepatic circulation the rate of synthesis will be high. Normally there are 1 to 2 g of bile salts in the enterohepatic circulation. If the transport process in the terminal ileum is functioning properly, only about 0.5 g is lost daily. Synthesis is regulated to replenish this loss.

Although cholic and chenodeoxycholic acids are not the only bile acids secreted, they are the only ones synthesized by the liver. Secondary bile acids are produced in the intestine through the action of microorganisms on primary bile acids. The chief secondary acids are deoxycholic and lithocholic. These acids are absorbed in the terminal ileum along with the primary bile acids, taken up by the hepatocytes, conjugated with taurine and glycine, and secreted in the bile. Thus bile contains a mixture of primary and secondary bile acids. Cholic, chenodeoxycholic, and deoxycholic acids normally appear in a ratio of 4:4:2. Usually only a small amount of lithocholic acid is present.

Cholesterol and phospholipids (primarily lecithins) also are secreted by the hepatocytes. The exact mechanisms of secretion are not known; but secretion appears to depend, in part, upon the secretion of bile acids. The higher the rate of bile acid secretion, the higher is the rate of cholesterol and phospholipid secretion. Once secreted into the intestine along with the other components of bile, cholesterol and lecithin are mixed with and handled as ingested cholesterol and lecithin (see Chapter 11).

The primary bile pigment in humans, bilirubin, is derived largely from the metabolic breakdown of hemoglobin (Fig. 10-3). Most of the hemoglobin comes from aged red blood cells that are disposed of by cells of the reticuloendothelial system. In the reticuloendothelial cells, hemoglobin is split into hemin and globin. The hemin ring is opened and oxidized, and the iron is removed to form bilirubin, which is then transported in the blood from the cells of the reticuloendothelial system to the hepatocytes. In transit, bilirubin is bound tightly to plasma albumin; very little is free in the plasma. Hepatocytes possess the ability to extract bilirubin from blood, conjugate it with glucuronic acid, and secrete the conjugated product into the bile. Bilirubin uptake by the hepatocytes is mediated by an active anion transport system. This system is

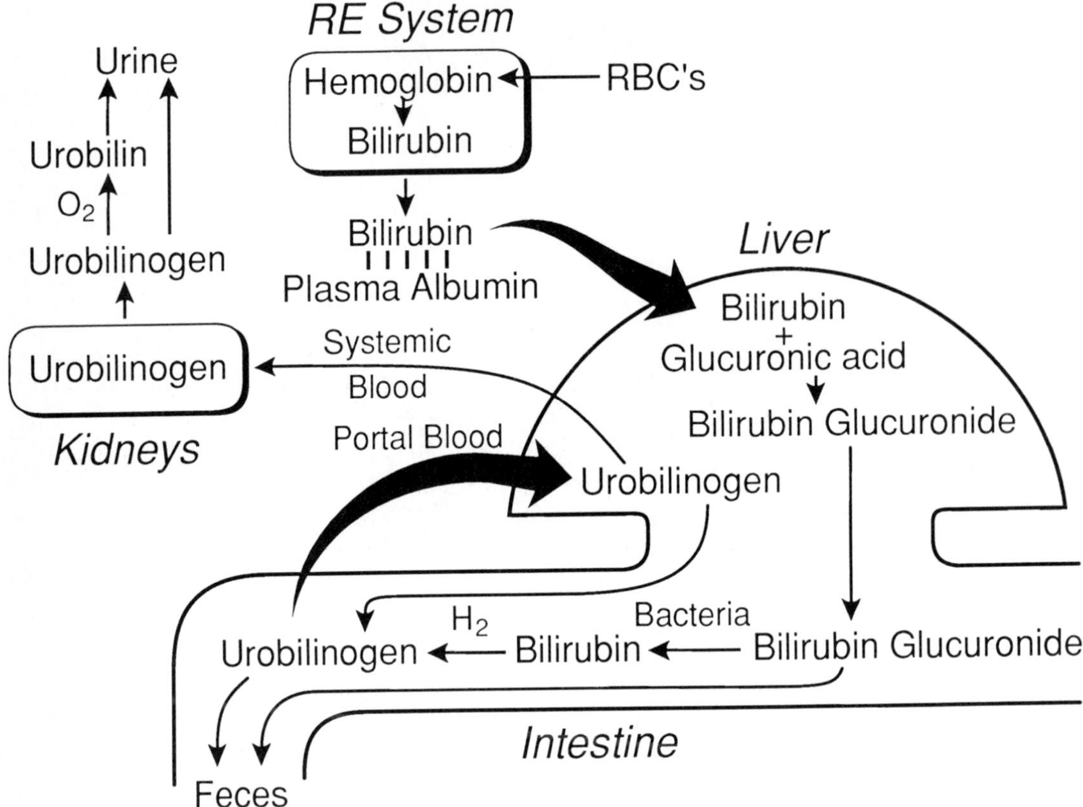

Fig. 10-3. Excretion of bile pigments. Bilirubin is produced by cells of the reticuloendothelial system from aged red blood cells. The unconjugated pigment is then carried, tightly bound to plasma albumin, to the liver. There it is actively taken up, conjugated with glucuronic acid, and secreted into the bile. The water-soluble conjugates are propelled along the intestine. In the distal small bowel and colon a portion of the conjugated pigment is acted upon by bacteria and becomes unconjugated bilirubin and other pigments. Some of these pigments are absorbed passively into the blood and either are returned to the liver and resecreted, or pass through the liver and are excreted by the kidneys. Most, however, pass through the colon and are excreted. *Bold arrows* indicate active absorption.

different from the one for active transport of bile acids but is shared by a number of other organic anions (e.g., sulfobromophthalein [Bromsulphalein, BSP] and various radiopaque dyes).

Bilirubin is not absorbed from the intestine in any appreciable amount. Some of the product, however, is altered in the bowel. Bacteria, primarily in the distal small bowel and colon, reduce bilirubin to urobilinogen, which is unconjugated. Some urobilinogen is excreted in the feces, but part is absorbed into the portal blood and returned to the liver. There most of the urobilinogen is extracted, conjugated, and secreted into the bile; however, some passes into the systemic circulation and is excreted by the kidneys. The urobilinogen is oxidized in the urine and feces to form urobilin and stercobilin, respectively. These pigments are in large part responsible

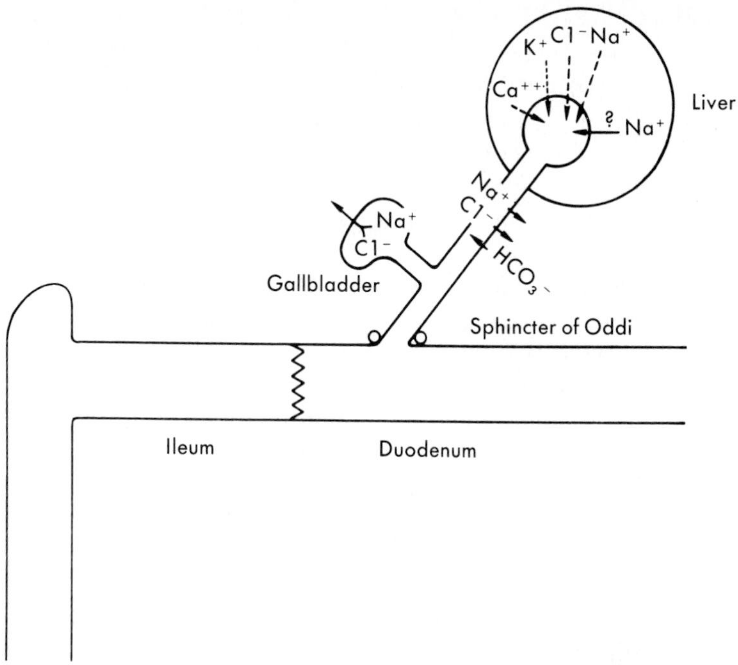

Fig. 10-4. Secretion and absorption of water and electrolytes. The osmotic gradient created by the active secretion of bile acids, and perhaps Na^+, causes water to move from the hepatocytes into the bile canaliculi. Ions accompany water movement, presumably via the process of bulk flow. Epithelial cells of the bile ducts are capable of actively absorbing Na^+ and Cl^- and of actively secreting Na^+ and HCO_3^-. In the gallbladder, salt absorption is accompanied by the absorption of water, thus concentrating the bile.

for the color of the excretory products of the body.

Two components of bile secretion have been identified. One is called "bile acid dependent." Bile acids, regardless of whether they are newly synthesized or extracted from the portal blood, are the major ions actively secreted by the hepatocytes. Their secretion, in turn, sets up an osmotic gradient down which water moves. The movement of water is accompanied by the passive movement of electrolytes (Fig. 10-4). The second component is called "bile acid independent secretion." There is evidence for the active transport of Na^+ by the hepatocytes. Also, as the canalicular bile flows through the bile ductules and ducts on its way to the gallbladder, its composition is altered (Fig. 10-4).

Both secretion and absorption take place in the ducts, secretion normally predominating. Bicarbonate is secreted actively by the epithelial cells that line the ducts. Absorption of water, Na^+, and Cl^- also can be demonstrated. The net effect of this secretory and absorptive activity is that the bile becomes more alkaline and its chloride content decreases. Secretory activity of the epithelial cells of the bile ductules and ducts is under hormonal control. Secretin stimulates production of bile that is relatively low in bile salt and high in HCO_3^- concentrations. It does this by increasing the active transport of sodium and bicarbonate from the epithelial cells into the bile.

BILE TRANSPORT TO AND STORAGE IN THE GALLBLADDER

The force responsible for flow of bile from the canaliculi toward the small intestine is primarily the secretory pressure generated by the hepatocytes and ductule epithelium. The hepatic end of the biliary tract is blind, being formed by the secretory cells of the liver. Thus as bile is secreted by these cells, pressure in the ducts rises. The active secretion of bile acids and electrolytes can make biliary secretory pressures reach 10 to 20 mm Hg.

Whether bile flows into the duodenum or into the gallbladder depends on a balance between the resistance to filling of the gallbladder and the resistance to flow through the terminal bile duct and sphincter of Oddi. The gallbladder is a distensible muscular organ that forms a blind outpouching of the biliary tract. Its inner surface is lined with a thin layer of epithelial cells having high absorptive capacities. The sphincter of Oddi is a thickening of the circular muscle of the bile duct located at the ductal entrance into the duodenum. Although this muscle is embedded in the wall of the duodenum it appears to be an entity separate from the duodenal musculature. Most of the time, during fasting, the gallbladder is readily distensible, and the sphincter of Oddi maintains closure of the terminal bile duct. Thus bile that is secreted by the liver flows into the gallbladder (Fig. 10-5, *A*).

The human gallbladder is not a large organ and when full can accommodate only 20 to 50 ml of fluid. During fasting, however, many times that volume of fluid may be secreted by the liver. The discrepancy between the amount of bile secreted by the liver and the amount stored in the gallbladder is accounted for by the gallbladder's ability to concentrate bile. The concentration of bile salts, bile pigments, and other large water-soluble molecules may increase 5 to 20 times as a result of water and electrolyte absorption.

Absorption of water and electrolytes is partly an active process. Na^+ absorption can occur against an electrochemical gradient, is a saturable process, depends upon metabolic activity, and demonstrates other characteristics of an active transport mechanism. Unlike the transport mechanisms for Na^+ that exist in other epithelia, however, transport in the gallbladder is not associated with the generation of any measurable electrical potential difference. In addition, it is highly dependent upon the presence of either Cl^- or HCO_3^-. Thus it appears as if Na^+ transport is coupled with the transport of an anion and is electrically neutral.

As in other epithelia, water movement in the gallbladder is dependent upon the active absorption of NaCl and $NaHCO_3$ and thus is entirely passive. The rows of epithelial cells of the mucosa have large lateral intercellular spaces near the basal membrane and possess tight junctions at their apices. Solute is transported actively from the cells into the intercellular space at the apical ends. This movement is then followed by the passive diffusion of H_2O. The movement of water molecules, however, is such that an osmotic gradient is set up in the intercellular spaces. The solution is hypertonic at the apical end and isotonic at the basal end. In the steady state this standing osmotic gradient is maintained and accounts for the absorption of a solution with fixed osmolality (see Fig. 12-5).

Absorption of Na^+, Cl^-, HCO_3^-, and H_2O influences the concentrations of other solutes in the bile. Ions such as K^+ and Ca^{++} become more concentrated. The concentration of micelles also increases during the absorption of water and electrolytes. The presence of micelles, which are known to have minimal osmotic activity, permits the high concentration of electrolytes, bile salts, phospholipids, and cholesterol to be isotonic in gallbladder bile.

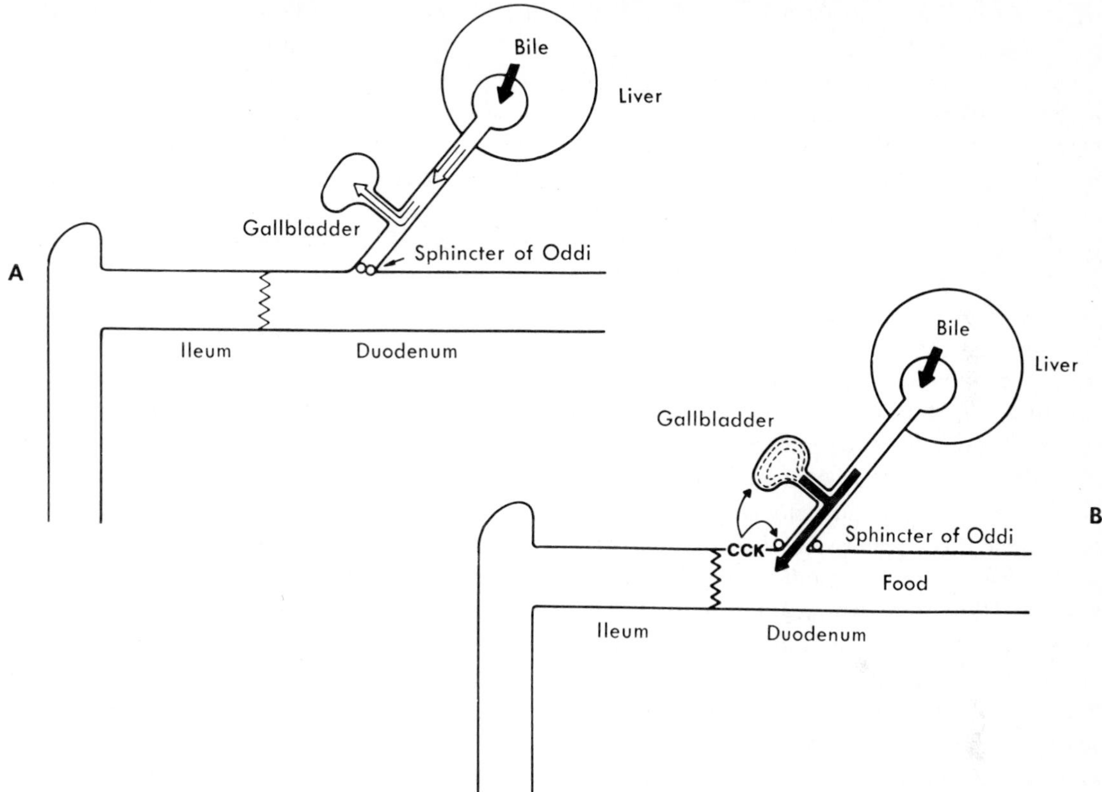

Fig. 10-5. A, Bile flow between periods of digestion. Bile is secreted continuously by the liver and flows toward the duodenum. In the interdigestive period the gallbladder is readily distensible and the sphincter of Oddi is contracted. Therefore bile flows into the gallbladder rather than into the duodenum. **B**, On eating, both hormonal (CCK) and neural stimuli cause contraction of the gallbladder and relaxation of the sphincter of Oddi. Thus bile flows into the bowel. Bile secretion by the liver increases as bile acids are returned via the enterohepatic circulation.

EXPULSION OF BILE AND TRANSPORT TO THE INTESTINE

Most bile secretion occurs during digestion of meals. However, significant amounts are secreted periodically during fasting in synchrony with the migrating motor complex (p. 45). The gallbladder contracts shortly before and during the period of intense sequential duodenal contractions. Thus bile, along with other secretions, is swept aborally along the bowel by these contractions. The stimuli responsible for coordinating gallbladder contraction with cyclical intestinal motility are not known.

Shortly after eating the gallbladder musculature contracts rhythmically and empties gradually (Fig. 10-5, *B*). The stimulus for its contraction appears to be primarily hormonal. Products of food digestion, particularly lipids, release cholecystokinin from the mucosa of the duodenum. This hormone is carried in the blood to the gallbladder, where it stimulates the musculature to contract. CCK is a potent stimulant of gallbladder muscle and appears to act directly. It is just as effective a stimulant to gallbladders that have been denervated either surgically or chemically. The role of other gastrointestinal hormones is less clear. Gastrin stimulates gallbladder contraction, but in doses that are well above the physiological range. Secretin appears to have little direct effect on the gallbladder though it may antagonize (or prevent) the effects of CCK.

Flow of bile from the gallbladder, through the common bile duct, and into the duodenum, is influenced by muscular activity of the common bile duct, the sphincter of Oddi, and the duodenum. The bile duct contains smooth muscle cells, and measurements of its contractile activity have been made in certain species. Some investigators maintain that peristaltic contractions of the duct do occur, and that these facilitate movement of bile into the duodenum. The relative importance of this mechanism is not known.

The sphincter of Oddi is a muscular ring surrounding the opening of the bile duct in the wall of the duodenum. Its relative contributions to the regulation of bile flow are sometimes difficult to assess because its own activity is influenced by the musculature of the duodenum. The sphincter can maintain closure of the bile duct independent of activity of the duodenal musculature. When the duodenum is relaxed, pressures of 12 to 30 mm Hg are needed to force fluid through a closed sphincter. However, bile flow through an open sphincter of Oddi is influenced markedly by the contractile activity of the duodenum. Bile enters an actively contracting bowel in spurts during periods of duodenal relaxation and stops during periods of contraction. The sphincter, like the muscle of the gallbladder, is controlled by the hormone CCK. In contrast to its action on the gallbladder, CCK relaxes the sphincter of Oddi and thereby allows bile to enter the duodenum.

The role of the autonomic nervous system in the control of bile flow is not clear. Stimulation of parasympathetic nerves causes an increase in bile flow and contraction of the gallbladder. Stimulation of sympathetic nerves has the opposite effect. Bile flow begins shortly after eating and may be part of the cephalic phase of digestion. The emotional state of the individual also has been shown to influence bile flow.

CLINICAL APPLICATIONS

Abnormalities of bile secretion can result from functional changes in the liver, bile ducts, gallbladder, and intestine. Because many of the components of bile are synthesized and/or actively secreted by hepatocytes, metabolic abnormalities of these cells can result in decreased bile production and increased plasma levels of those constituents normally excreted in the bile (e.g., bile acids and pigments). Metabolic abnormalities more commonly result from the destruction of hepatocytes by infectious agents (e.g., viral hepatitis) and by various toxins. There are, however, several conditions characterized by genetic deficiencies in one or more of the steps of bilirubin secretion. These deficiencies also can result in jaundice (a visually detectable buildup of bile pigments in the blood).

Besides the rather striking changes in hepatocyte function seen with hepatocyte destruction and genetic defects, subtle changes also can produce pathological conditions. In many individuals the quantity of bile produced by the liver may be normal but the quality abnormal. To be stable, bile must contain certain proportions of bile salts, phospholipids, and cholesterol. If there is a relative excess of cholesterol it may precipitate to form gallstones. Some 10% of the white population over 29 years of age in the United States is estimated to have gallstones.

Abnormalities of the bile ducts and gallbladder are usually secondary to the processes of obstruction (e.g., stones or tumor) and/or infection. Obstruction can result in severe pain and can lead to reflux of bile into the liver parenchyma and eventually the systemic circulation. Bacterial infections, often occurring secondary to stones, also can initiate and/or perpetuate stone formation. Several strains of bacteria (such as *Escherichia coli*) produce β-glucuronidase, which deconjugates conjugated bile pigments. These unconjugated pigments, which are less soluble, will then precipitate to form pigment stones or a nidus for precipitation of cholesterol.

Abnormalities of intestinal function can alter the secretion of products that undergo enterohepatic circulation. For example, if the terminal ileum is diseased or removed, bile salt absorption is reduced. This decreases the bile salt pool (and hence bile salt secretion) and increases synthesis of bile acids by the liver. In addition, bile acids that enter the colon induce water secretion by the colonic mucosa and cause diarrhea.

CLINICAL TESTS

The major tests of bile secretion revolve around the measurement of serum levels of endogenous substances normally secreted in the bile, the measurement of secretion of exogenous substances injected into the blood, and the x-ray visualization of the biliary tract.

Plasma levels of both bile salts and bile pigments are elevated in many types of hepatobiliary disease. Of these substances, bilirubin is the most commonly measured entity.

Abnormalities in hepatic function often can be detected before the elevation of serum bilirubin and the development of jaundice. This is done by intravenously injecting chemicals such as sulfobromophthalein and indocyanine green. These substances normally are taken up and secreted by the same anionic transport system utilized for the hepatic secretion of bile pigments. Impairment of hepatocyte function is characterized by a slower than normal disappearance of these injected substances from the blood.

X-ray visualization of the biliary tract is the most common mode of detecting gallstones. Many of the stones are radiopaque and are visualized on a standard film. Others, however, are radiolucent and thus not obvious. A radiopaque dye is required to facilitate visualization of these stones. The dye usually consists of iodinated anions that are taken up and secreted by the anionic transport system of the hepatocytes. The stones are then surrounded by the dye and appear as holes in the contrast medium. Radiopaque dyes are effective only if the anionic transport system of the hepatocytes is functional; therefore the tests do not work in the presence of jaundice.

SUGGESTED REFERENCES

Erlinger S: Physiology of bile secretion and enterohepatic circulation. In Johnson LR, editor: Physiology of the gastrointestinal tract, New York, 1987, Raven Press.

Forker EL: Mechanisms of hepatic bile formation, Ann Rev Physiol 39:323-347, 1977.

Rose RC: Absorptive functions of the gallbladder. In Johnson LR, editor: Physiology of the gastrointestinal tract, New York, 1987, Raven Press.

Scharschmidt BF: Bile formation and gallbladder and bile duct function. In Sleisenger MH and Fordtran JS, editors: Gastrointestinal disease, Philadelphia, 1983, WB Saunders Co.

11 Digestion and Absorption

Gilbert A. Castro

The physiological principles presented in this chapter explain how food is broken down into small absorbable molecules and how these products are transported into the blood. Factors that regulate or alter the processes are considered. These processes result in the energy-yielding substrates and precursors for the biosynthetic reactions of the body.

STRUCTURAL-FUNCTIONAL ASSOCIATIONS

Food assimilation takes place primarily in the small intestine and is aided by anatomical modifications that increase the luminal surface area—Kerkring's folds, villi, and microvilli. The microvilli are prominent on the apical surface of columnar epithelial cells or enterocytes and occur to a lesser extent on goblet cells. Collectively the microvillous region comprises the brush border.

Several cell types make up the intestinal epithelium. Students of digestive and absorptive physiology are most familiar with enterocytes and goblet cells. Enterocytes function in digestion, absorption, and secretion. Goblet cells secrete mucus. The function of mucus is not clear but may be related to physical, chemical, and immunological protection. Both enterocytes and goblet cells are derived from a common stem cell within the intestinal crypts. Enterocytes and goblet cells become differentiated as they move upward from the base of the crypt, and their characteristics are expressed more strongly as they migrate farther up the villus. As they reach the tip of the villus the cells are extruded and become a component of the succus entericus. In humans the time needed to replace the entire population of epithelial cells (the cell turnover time) is 3 to 6 days. Cell proliferation, differentiation, and maturation are partly controlled by gastrointestinal hormones and partly influenced by conditions such as starvation, irradiation, or partial bowel resection. Despite the interplay between a basic dynamic process and the extrinsic factors that affect epithelial development, the mucosal appearance remains relatively constant.

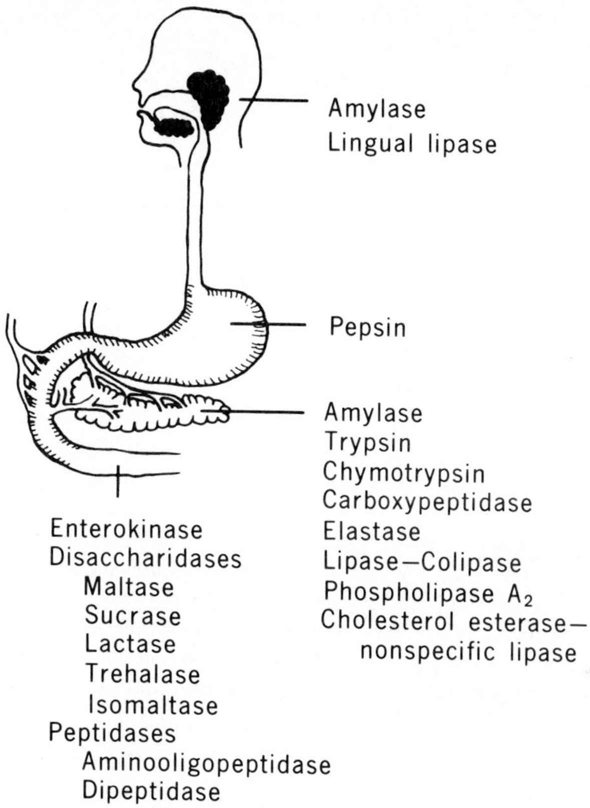

Fig. 11-1. Source of the principal luminal and membrane-bound digestive enzymes.

DIGESTION

Digestion is the chemical breakdown of food by enzymes secreted by glandular cells in the mouth, chief cells in the stomach, and the exocrine cells of the pancreas, or bound to the apical membranes of enterocytes. Although some digestion of carbohydrates, proteins, and fats takes place in the stomach, the final breakdown of these substances occurs in the small intestine.

The enzymes important in digestion are summarized in Fig. 11-1. Luminal or cavital digestion is due to enzymes secreted by the salivary glands, stomach, and pancreas. Significant chemical degradation of food is carried out, also, by hydrolytic enzymes associated with the small intestinal brush border. Hydrolysis by these enzymes is termed "contact" or "membrane" digestion. "Membrane digestion" is a more acceptable term, because "contact digestion" connotes activity by exogenous enzymes that become adsorbed on the epithelial surface. "Membrane digestion" implies hydrolysis by enzymes synthesized by epithelial cells and inserted into the apical membrane as integral components. The half-life of membrane-bound enzymes (such as oligosaccharidases) is less than that of epithelial cells. Thus breakdown and resynthesis occur several times during the life of a single cell.

Digestion and absorption of essentially all major dietary products take place in the small intestine. Despite the degradation of colonic contents by bacteria, physiologically impor-

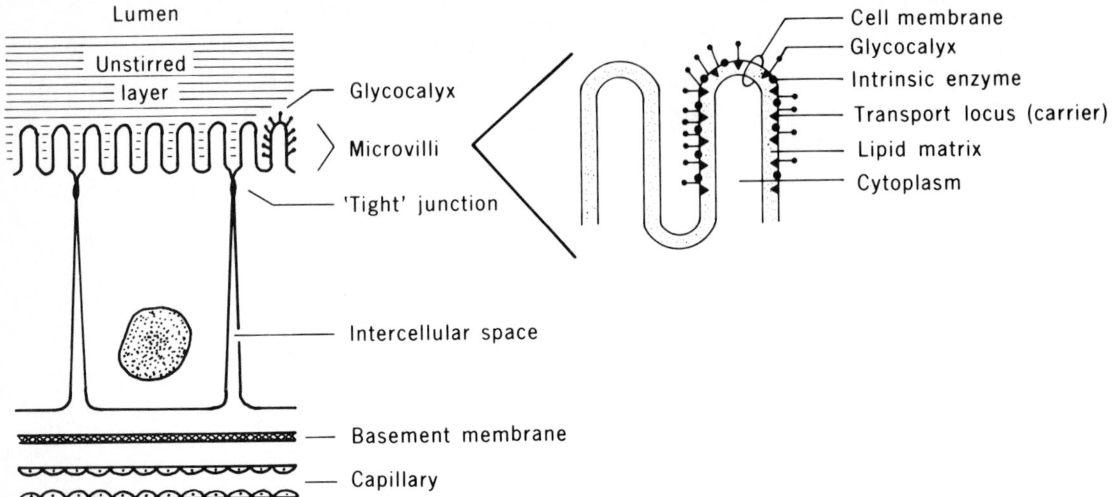

Fig. 11-2. Mucosal barrier. Solutes moving across the enterocyte from the intestinal lumen to the blood must traverse an unstirred layer of fluid, a glycocalyx, the apical membrane, cytoplasm of the cell, basolateral cell membrane, the basement membrane, and finally the wall of the capillary or lymphatic vessel. Microvilli are morphological modifications of the cell membrane that comprise the brush border. The importance of this region in digestion and absorption of nutrients is depicted by the enlarged microvillus, which illustrates the spatial arrangement of enzymes and carrier molecules.

tant digestion does not occur in the colon. Nonetheless, absorption in this organ is impressive. A practical illustration is that some medications administered as rectal suppositories are systemically functional. During health the principal substances absorbed from the colon are water and electrolytes. However, life is possible without this organ, as evidenced by patients who thrive after colectomy.

ABSORPTION

Although the brush border is the site of activity for a number of digestive enzymes, it is also the barrier that must be traversed by nutrients, water, and electrolytes on the way to the blood or lymph. The terms "transport" and "absorption" often are used interchangeably to mean the movement of materials from the intestinal lumen into the blood. "Secretion" implies movement in the opposite direction.

Mucosal Membrane

Conceptually the plasma membrane of the enterocyte often is considered the only factor restricting the free movement of substances from the gut lumen into the blood or lymph. However, transmural movement actually takes place over a complex pathway. This is conveyed schematically in Fig. 11-2 and includes (1) an unstirred layer of fluid, (2) the glycocalyx ("fuzzy coat") covering the microvilli, (3) the cell membrane, (4) the cytoplasm of the enterocyte, (5) the basal or lateral cell membrane, (6) the intercellular space, (7) the basement membrane, and (8) the membrane of the capillary or lymph vessel.

Transport Processes

An outstanding property of the enterocyte membrane is its capacity to control the flux of solutes and fluid between the lumen and blood. This involves several mechanisms. Pinocytosis occurs at the base of microvilli and may be a major mechanism in the uptake of protein. Other uptake processes include passive diffusion, facilitated diffusion, and active transport. In the case of passive diffusion, the epithelium behaves like an inert barrier and the particles traverse this cell layer through pores in the cell membrane or through intercellular spaces. The tight junction between apposing enterocytes (Fig. 11-2) forms a mechanical seal that prevents mixing of interstitial fluid with luminal contents. This seal, however, is relatively leaky to ions and water in certain regions of the intestine, allowing some exchange between the lumen and intercellular spaces.

ADAPTATION OF DIGESTIVE AND ABSORPTIVE PROCESSES

Alterations in intestinal functions in response to a variety of factors are well documented. Functional adjustments that maintain homeostasis or allow an animal to cope better with its environment are termed "adaptations." The quality and degree of adjustment are dependent upon the type of environmental stimulus encountered. Clinical situations in which the capacity to adapt is magnified are small-bowel resection and bypass. Until recently physicians knew only that a patient subjected to one of these operations underwent an initial phase of undernutrition, steatorrhea, and acidic diarrhea and that these symptoms tended to be alleviated with time. Relief from the symptoms is believed to be attributable to adaptations. For example, after proximal bowel resection or bypass the remaining segment undergoes hyperplastic changes accompanied by enhancement of particular absorptive and digestive functions. Adaptation is limited in some circumstances. This point is illustrated by the fact that the absorption of vitamin B_{12} and bile salts is confined strictly to the terminal ileum. Other regions of the GI tract cannot compensate if the absorptive capacity for these compounds in the ileum is lost.

In certain genetic abnormalities, such as lactase deficiency, the capacity to adapt is lost. This condition, as well as pancreatic and intestinal diseases of varied etiology, contributes to maldigestion and malabsorption.

CARBOHYDRATE ASSIMILATION

Principal Dietary Forms

The average daily intake of carbohydrates in the United States is about 300 g. Starch comprises about 50% of the total, sucrose about 30%, lactose 6%, and maltose 1% to 2%. Trehalose, glucose, fructose, sorbitol, cellulose, hemicellulose, and pectins make up most of the remainder. Starch is a high–molecular weight compound consisting of two polysaccharides, amylose and amylopectin. Amylose is a straight-chain polymer of glucose linked by α-1,4 glycosidic bonds. The repeating disaccharide unit is maltose. Amylopectin is similar to amylose; however, in addition to 1,4-linkages there are 1,6-linkages for every 20 to 30 glucose units. Glycogen is a high–molecular weight polysaccharide similar to amylopectin in molecular structure but having considerably more 1,6-linkages. Maltose and trehalose are dimers of glucose in 1,4- and 1,1-linkages, respectively. Sucrose is a disaccharide consisting of 1 mol of glucose bound at the number 1 carbon to the number 2 carbon of fructose. Lactose is 1 mol of galactose bound at the number 1 carbon to the number 4 carbon of glucose in a β-linkage.

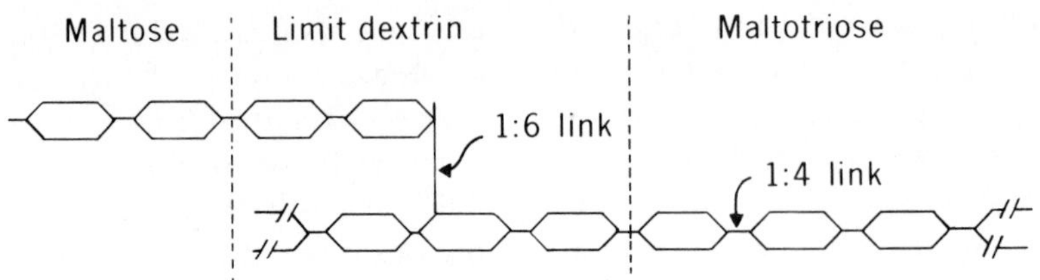

Fig. 11-3. Products of starch hydrolysis by α-amylase.

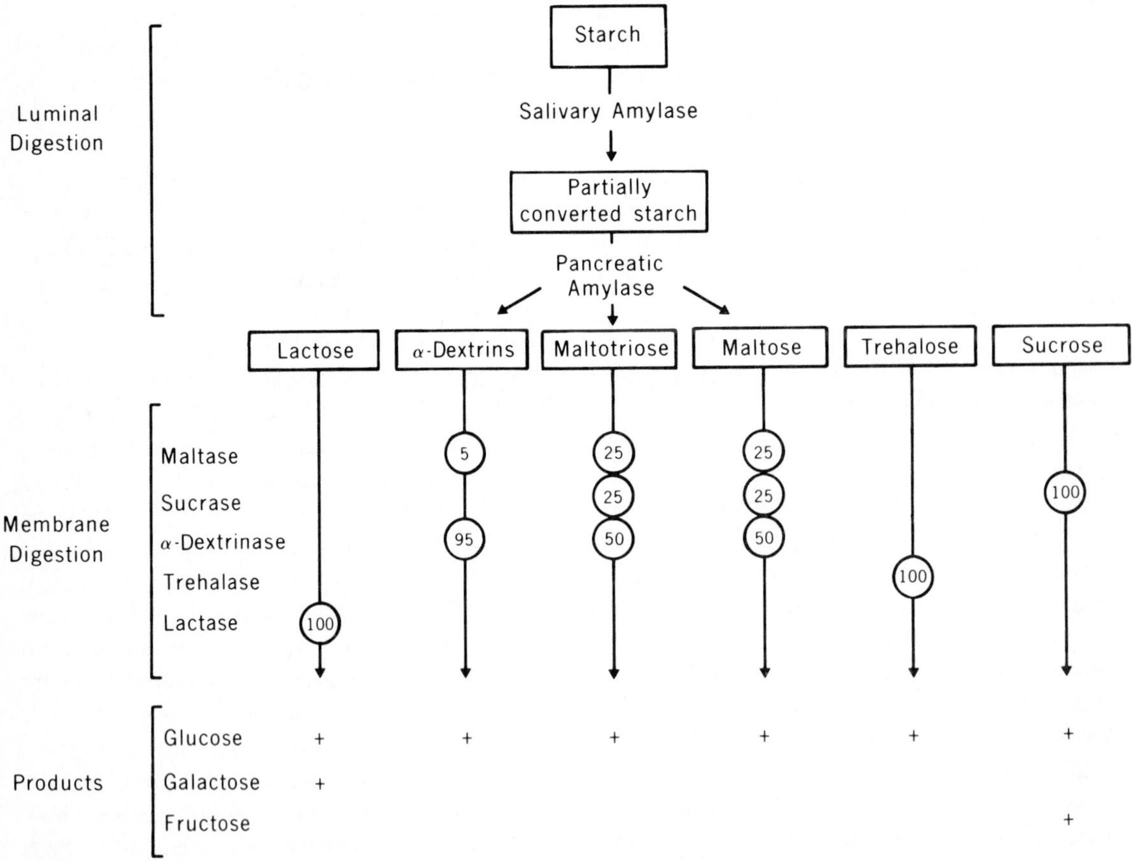

Luminal Digestion

Starch
Salivary Amylase
Partially converted starch
Pancreatic Amylase

Membrane Digestion

	Lactose	α-Dextrins	Maltotriose	Maltose	Trehalose	Sucrose
Maltase		5	25	25		
Sucrase			25	25		100
α-Dextrinase		95	50	50		
Trehalase					100	
Lactase	100					

Products

	Lactose	α-Dextrins	Maltotriose	Maltose	Trehalose	Sucrose
Glucose	+	+	+	+	+	+
Galactose	+					
Fructose						+

Fig. 11-4. Summary of the luminal digestion of starch and the membrane digestion of disaccharides and oligosaccharides. Brush border enzymes are listed in decreasing order of activity. The specific activity of lactase is generally only about 5% as great as maltase activity. *Circled numbers* denote the substrate specificity of human brush border saccharidases. For example, maltose and maltotriose are hydrolyzed by three different enzymes. Glucose and galactose are absorbed by a carrier system that can be energized to transport actively, and fructose is taken up by facilitated diffusion.

Digestion

The human GI tract does not possess cellulases capable of digesting β-glucose linkages of cellulose and hemicellulose. Thus these carbohydrates represent undigestable fiber. Luminal digestion of starch begins in the mouth with the action of salivary α-amylase and ends in the small intestine through the action of pancreatic α-amylase. Human salivary and pancreatic amylases have optimum activities near neutral pH and are activated by Cl^-. Although salivary amylase is destroyed by acid in the stomach, some enzymatic activity occurs within the bolus of food. Most starch digestion, however, occurs in the small intestine. Hydrolysis occurs not only in the lumen but also at the surface of epithelial cells because some amylase is adsorbed to the brush border.

Amylase attacks only the interior α-1,4-bonds of amylose, yielding maltose and the trisaccharide maltotriose. Hydrolysis of amylopectin and glycogen yields similar products plus α-limit dextrins (Fig. 11-3). The latter are oligosaccharides of glucose, formed because the α-1,6-linkages are resistant to enzymatic attack.

Products of amylase action on starch and other major dietary sugars are hydrolyzed by brush border carbohydrases. Several brush border enzymes hydrolyze more than one substrate (Fig. 11-4). The 1,6-bonds of limit dextrins are hydrolyzed by α-dextrinase (isomaltase) and maltase. Maltase, sucrase, and α-dextrinase hydrolyze maltose and maltotriose to glucose. Sucrase, lactase, and trehalase break down sucrose, lactose, and trehalose, respectively.

Sucrase and isomaltase occur together as a molecular complex. The fact that congenital deficiencies of sucrase and α-dextrinase occur together reveals a close functional relationship between these two enzymes. In humans, sucrase-dextrinase is a compound molecule, one unit with absolute specificity for sucrose and one for the α-1,6-linkage of a α-limit dextrin.

In general there is a large disaccharidase reserve in the small intestine, so much that the rate-limiting step in sugar assimilation is not digestion but the absorption of free hexoses following hydrolysis. Under normal circumstances the major portion of sugar assimilation is complete in the proximal jejunum.

Absorption of Digestion Products

For the body to utilize food-derived monosaccharides, they must be absorbed. Fig. 11-5 shows how glucose absorption from the intestine occurs by passive as well as active processes. Although there are aqueous channels between enterocytes and pores in brush border membranes, dietary hexoses are too large to penetrate the membranes in any significant degree by passive diffusion. In humans the major route of entry into enterocytes is by brush border membrane carrier systems.

Fructose is transported by facilitated diffusion. In some animals it is metabolized partly to glucose, which in turn enters the circulation as it leaves the enterocytes. In humans such metabolism is minimal.

The carrier systems for fructose and glucose-galactose differ insofar as the fructose carrier cannot be energized for active transport, whereas the glucose carrier can. Glucose and galactose are absorbed by secondary active transport via a Na^+-dependent carrier system (Fig. 11-6). Mutual inhibition of glucose or galactose transport by the presence of the other indicates that they are transported by a common carrier.

The glucose entry step depicted in Fig. 11-6 involves a carrier that binds sodium and glucose molecules; two Na^+ for each glucose molecule are transported into the cell. The entry step is only slightly reversible because of removal of intracellular Na^+ by the pump

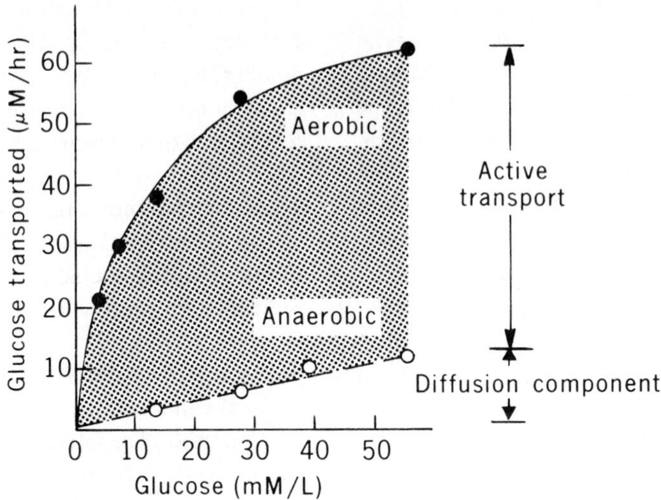

Fig. 11-5. Absorption rates of glucose from a solution perfused through the intestine of a guinea pig. In the absence of oxygen the rate of mediated uptake is proportional to concentration. When oxygen is available for cellular respiration the uptake is greater and the carrier system can be energized for active transport. *(Modified from Ricklis E and Quastel JH: Can J Biochem Physiol 36:348-362, 1958.)*

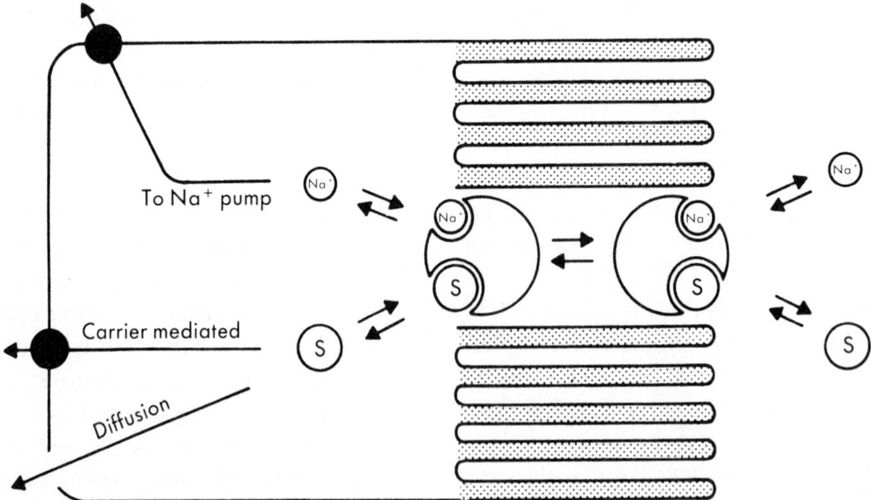

Fig. 11-6. Summary of a sodium-dependent carrier system for glucose-galactose. Absorption involves the rapid movement from lumen to blood by an entry step and exit step mediated by two separate carrier molecules with specificity for hexose. The system is energized by an ATP-dependent Na^+ pump that maintains sodium gradient favoring the entry of Na^+ into the cell, with the concomitant cotransport of substrate, *S*. When Na^+ is pumped from the cell, more Na^+ and glucose are transported into the cell from the lumen. The transport capacity of the carrier involved in glucose exit appears to equal that involved in glucose entry, because glucose does not accumulate within the cells to a large degree.

on the basolateral membrane. Energy input (ATP) drives the sodium pump and maintains a Na^+ gradient favoring glucose entry. Inhibition of the Na^+ with specific chemicals (such as ouabain) or interference in cellular energy production leads to cytosolic accumulation of Na^+ and the abolition of active sugar transport. The exit of glucose from the cytosol into the intracellular space is attributed partly to diffusion but mostly to the presence of a sodium-independent carrier located at the basolateral membrane.

Regulation of Absorption

The capacity of the human small intestine to absorb free sugars is enormous. It has been estimated that hexoses equivalent to 22 pounds of sucrose could be absorbed daily. There appears to be little physiological control of sugar absorption. However, chemoreceptors and osmoreceptors in the proximal small intestine control the motility and emptying of the stomach through a negative feedback process mediated by hormones and neural reflexes. As an example, a volume of isotonic citrate solution of 750 ml placed in the human stomach passes into the small bowel in 20 minutes. The volume delivered in the same time is reduced if sucrose or glucose is added to the citrate solution. The amount delivered is related inversely to the sugar concentration.

Abnormalities in Carbohydrate Assimilation

It is obvious from the foregoing consideration that polysaccharides and oligosaccharides are absorbed not as such but as monosaccharides. Carbohydrates remaining in the intestinal lumen increase the osmotic pressure of the luminal contents because of defects in digestion and absorption. Bacterial fermentation of these carbohydrates in the lower small intestine and colon adds to this osmotic effect. The osmotic retention of water in the lumen leads to diarrhea.

Diarrhea caused by the poor assimilation of dietary carbohydrates most commonly is caused by deficiencies in carbohydrate-splitting enzymes in the intestinal brush border. Lactase deficiency, the most frequently observed congenital disaccharidase deficiency (which may also be acquired in later life), can exist in the absence of any other intestinal malfunction. Intolerance of sucrose and isomaltose is a rare disease found primarily in children. Intolerance of maltose has not been documented. The observation that lactase deficiency is a relatively common genetic disease, while maltase deficiency is not, may be related to the fact that only one enzyme displays significant lactase activity, whereas several display activity against maltose (Fig. 11-4). Thus maltose intolerance would require the simultaneous absence of all enzymes possessing maltase activity. Maldigestion of starch in humans in nonexistent, because pancreatic amylase is secreted in tremendous excess.

Intolerance to glucose and galactose has been documented in rare instances. In these cases the patients thrive and show no symptoms when fed fructose. The explanation for this is found in the specificity of sugar absorption. Glucose and chemically related sugars are absorbed by a Na^+-dependent secondary active transport process, whereas fructose is absorbed by Na^+-independent facilitated diffusion. In these patients the carrier for glucose is absent.

Besides defects in carbohydrate assimilation caused by the congenital or acquired enzyme deficiencies, assimilation of dietary sugars may be impaired by diseases of the gastrointestinal tract. Celiac disease, certain bacterial infections, and some protozoan and helminth infections are associated with inflammation and structural derangements in the small bowel mucosa. These conditions often are at-

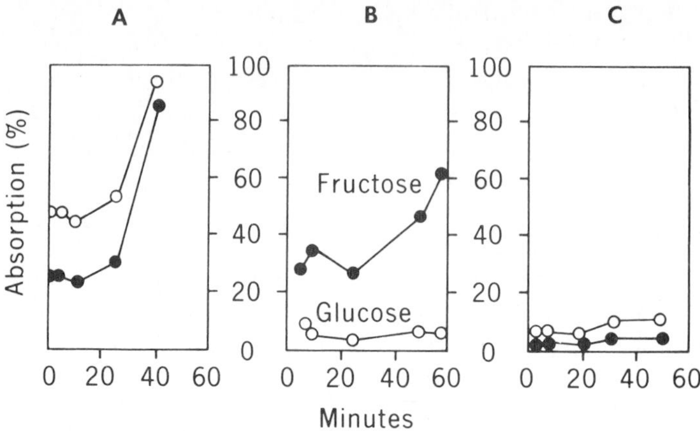

Fig. 11-7. Relative rates of absorption of fructose and glucose in an equimolar mixture studied by an intubation technique in, **A**, a control subject; **B**, a patient with glucose malabsorption; and **C**, a patient with celiac disease. *(From Dahlqvist A: In Sipple HL and McNutt KW, editors: Sugars in nutrition, New York, 1974, Academic Press, Inc.)*

tended by brush border enzyme deficiencies and hexose malabsorption (Fig. 11-7). It is not uncommon to find lactase deficiency as a long-term consequence of intestinal disease, because this enzyme is present in the intestine at low levels compared to maltase and sucrase (see Fig. 11-4).

Symptoms of osmotic diarrhea include cramps and abdominal distention. An oral tolerance test can be used to diagnose disaccharidase deficiency if this is a suspected cause. After an overnight fast, adult patients are fed 50 g of lactose in a 10% aqueous solution (children are usually fed 2 g/kg body weight). Blood samples are taken for glucose analysis before and at 5, 10, 15, 30, 45, and 60 minutes after lactose administration. An increase in blood glucose of at least 25 mg/100 ml over fasted levels indicates normal hydrolysis of lactose and normal absorption of the glucose product. A flat lactose tolerance curve or failure to observe a rise in blood glucose over 25 mg/100 ml following lactose ingestion indicates low lactase activity. A value between 20 and 25 mg/100 ml is questionable. In this case the test may be repeated; or, if laboratory facilities permit, intestinal biopsy specimens can be collected and examined for enzyme activity. In dealing with biopsy specimens, enzyme activity usually is expressed as units per gram of tissue protein. Tolerance tests for disaccharides other than lactose are seldom performed, but a similar procedure would suffice. Glucose or galactose tolerance tests should be performed to exclude monosaccharide malabsorption as the cause of a flat lactose tolerance curve.

PROTEIN ASSIMILATION

Digestion

Protein digestion begins in the stomach with the action of pepsin. The enzyme precursor, pepsinogen, is secreted by chief cells in response to a meal and low gastric pH. Acid in the stomach is responsible for activating pepsinogen to pepsin. Three pepsin isozymes have been recognized. All have a pH optimum of 1 to 3 and are denatured above pH 5. Pep-

Table 11-1 Principal pancreatic proteases

Enzyme	Primary action
Endopeptidases	Hydrolyze interior peptide bonds of polypeptides and proteins.
Trypsin	Attacks peptide bonds involving basic amino acids; yields products with basic amino acids at C-terminal end
Chymotrypsin	Attacks peptide bonds involving aromatic amino acids, leucine, glutamine, and methionine; yields peptide products with these amino acids at C-terminal end
Elastase	Attacks peptide bonds involving neutral aliphatic amino acids; yields products with neutral amino acids at C-terminal end.
Exopeptidases	Hydrolyze external peptide bonds of polypeptides and protein.
Carboxypeptidase A	Attacks peptides with aromatic and neutral aliphatic amino acids at C-terminal end
Carboxypeptidase B	Attacks peptides with basic amino acids at C-terminal end

sin is an endopeptidase with specificity for peptide bonds involving aromatic L-amino acids.

Pepsin activity terminates when the gastric contents mix with alkaline pancreatic juice in the small bowel. Food in the intestine stimulates the release of secretin and CCK, which in turn causes the pancreas to secrete bicarbonate and enzymes into the intestinal lumen.

There are two general classes of pancreatic proteases, endopeptidases and exopeptidases. The basis of classification and the particular characteristics of specific enzymes belonging to each class are given in Table 11-1.

Pancreatic proteases are secreted into the duodenum as inactive precursors. Trypsinogen, which lacks proteolytic activity, is activated by enterokinase, an enzyme located on the brush border of duodenal enterocytes. The exact chemical composition of enterokinase is not known; however, the fact that the molecule is 41% carbohydrate probably prevents its rapid digestion by proteolytic enzymes. Enterokinase activates trypsinogen by releasing a hexapeptide from the N-terminal end of the precursor molecule (Fig. 11-8). Active trypsin, once formed, acts autocatalytically in the manner of enterokinase to activate the bulk of trypsinogen. Trypsin also activates other peptidase precursors from the pancreas (Fig. 11-8). Chymotrypsinogen is activated by cleavage of the peptide bond between arginine and isoleucine, which are the fifteenth and sixteenth amino acid residues at the N-terminus. Although structural rearrangement occurs, no peptide fragment is released because of a disulfide bond between the cysteine residues at positions 1 and 122 in the protein chain. This configuration is the active form of chymotrypsinogen. Cleavage at other points in the chymotrypsinogen molecule produces other molecular species of chymotrypsin having relatively little physiological importance. The exact mechanism for activation of proelastase is not known and activation of procarboxypeptidases A and B is relatively complicated, involving proteolysis of at least two proenzymes.

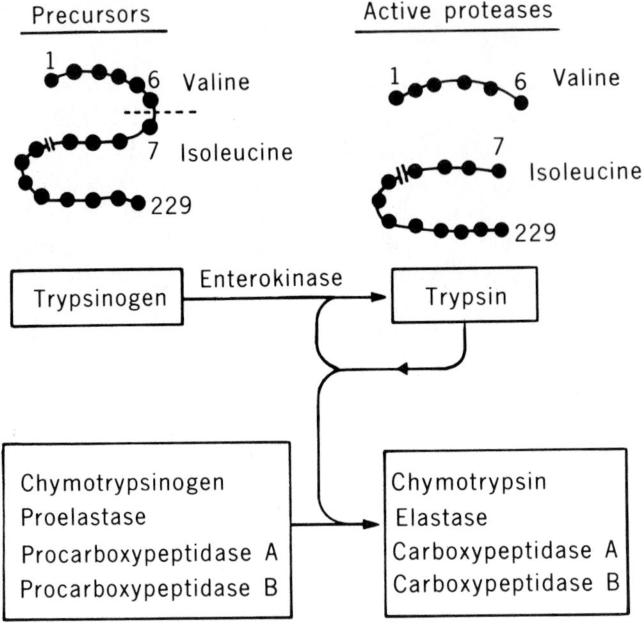

Fig. 11-8. Activation of pancreatic proteolytic enzymes.

Once in the small intestine, pancreatic enzymes undergo rapid inactivation because of autodigestion. Trypsin is the enzyme primarily responsible for inactivation.

Absorption of Digestion Products

Membrane digestion and absorption are closely related phenomena in protein assimilation, and physiologists have been occupied by two fundamental questions concerning them: (1) In what form do products of proteolysis cross the brush border membrane of the epithelial cell? (2) In what form do these products leave the cell to enter the blood?

L-Isomers of amino acids are absorbed by carrier-mediated mechanisms in much the same manner as glucose is absorbed. As with glucose the cell entry process requires Na^+ as part of a ternary complex (see Fig. 11-6), and uphill transfer occurs by secondary active transport.

Certain L-amino acids compete with one another for uptake by intestinal cells. Studies of competition have led to the recognition of several different carrier systems for amino acid absorption (Table 11-2). There is little doubt that the absorption of free amino acids by gut mucosa is physiologically important. However, amino acids appear in portal blood faster and reach a higher level when peptides from an acid hydrolysate of protein contact the gut mucosa than when there is an equimolar solution of free amino acid (Fig. 11-9). Also, greater amounts of total nitrogen are absorbed from a solution of trypsin hydrolysate of proteins than from an equivalent solution of amino acids in free form. Competition for transport between two chemically related amino acids is not observed when the same two acids are absorbed after ingestion of their dipeptides and tripeptides. In addition, the site in the intestine for the maximum absorption of amino acids in small peptide form is different from that for the absorption of free

Table 11-2 Carrier systems for the transport of amino acids

Type*	Examples of acids transported
Neutral (α-amino-monocarboxylic)	Aromatic (tryptophan, phenylalanine, tyrosine) Aliphatic (glycine,† alanine, serine, threonine, valine, leucine, isoleucine) Histidine, methionine, asparagine, glutamine, cysteine, proline,† hydroxyproline†
Basic (cationic)	Lysine, arginine, ornithine, cystine
Acidic (anionic)	Glutamic acid, asparatic acid
"Imino"‡	Proline,† hydroxyproline,† γ-amino butyric acid, taurine, glycine,† other amino acids with amino group in β and γ positions

*Categorization is based on specificity for L-stereoisomers, the position of the amino group relative to the carboxyl group, and the presence of secondary amino or carboxyl groups.
†Amino acids transported by more than one system.
‡The term "imino" acid is considered a misnomer, because various amino acid types may be transported by this system.

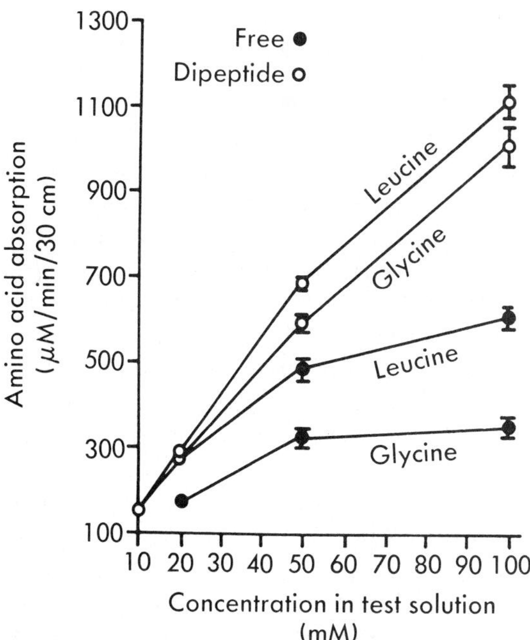

Fig. 11-9. Jejunal rates of glycine and leucine absorption (mean ± SEM, five subjects) from perfusion of test solutions containing either L-glycyl-L-leucine or an equimolar mixture of free L-glycine and free L-leucine. *(From Adibi SA: J Clin Invest 50:2266-2275, 1971.)*

amino acid. The current explanation of these findings is that a separate carrier system for small peptides is involved in absorption. For example, free glycine absorption requires an amino acid carrier system. If saturation of the system occurs under physiological conditions, the maximum rate of uptake becomes limiting. If, however, a second carrier for dipeptides or tripeptides of glycine is present, the amino acids can enter the cell in small-peptide form. Thus two separate systems for glycine entry exist and work in parallel.

The prevailing concepts regarding protein assimilation are illustrated in Fig. 11-10. Luminal digestion of a protein meal produces free amino acids and small peptides. As with the free acids, dipeptides and tripeptides resulting from digestion can be absorbed intact by carrier-mediated processes. However, tetra-, penta-, and hexapeptides are poorly absorbed; instead they are hydrolyzed by brush border peptidases to free amino acids or smaller absorbable peptides. The number and degree of specificity of peptide carriers are unclear but are definitely different from those of carriers that transport free amino acids.

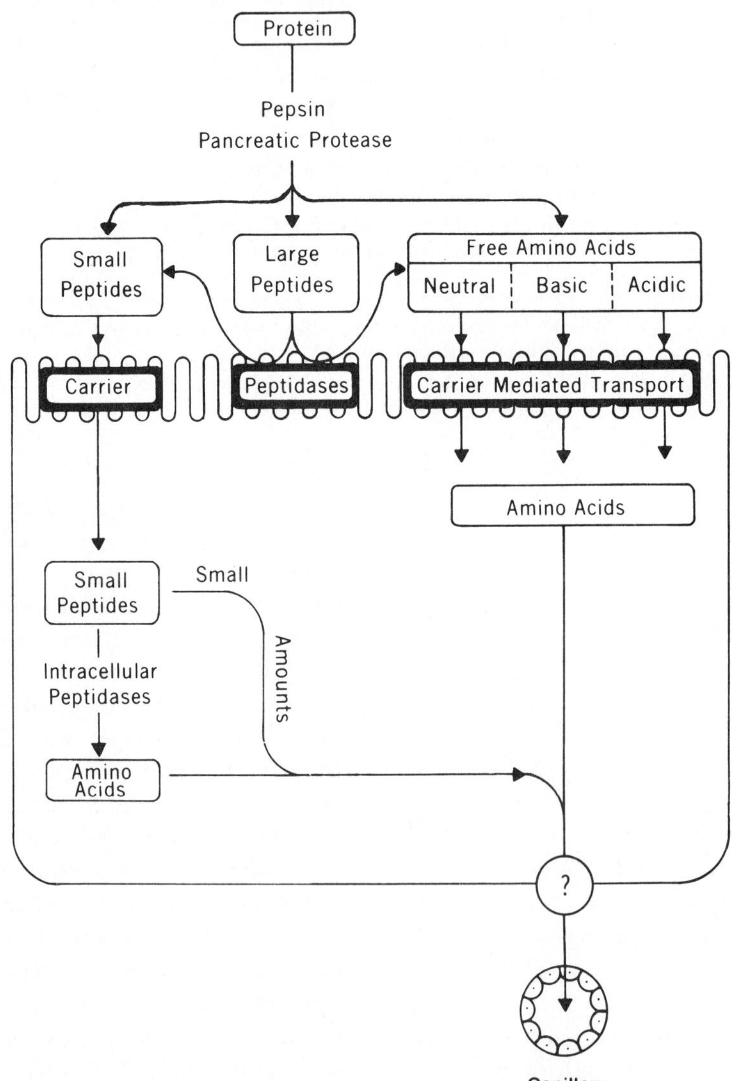

Fig. 11-10. Summary of digestion and absorption of dietary protein. Approximately one-third of the total amino acid is absorbed in free form after luminal digestion. The remaining is absorbed as free acid or dipeptide and tripeptide following membrane digestive processes.

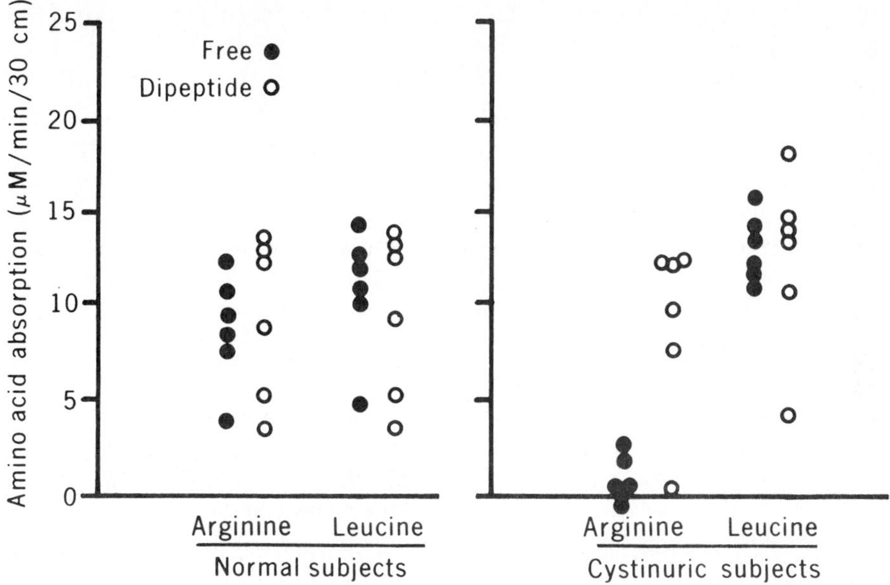

Fig. 11-11. Jejunal absorption of free arginine and leucine during perfusion of solutions containing L-arginine (1 mM) and L-leucine (1 mM) or L-arginyl-L-leucine (1 mM). Results are from studies carried out in six normal subjects and six cystinuric patients. *(From Silk DBA and Dawson AM: In Crane RK and Guyton AC, editors: International review of physiology. III, Gastrointestinal physiology, Baltimore, 1979, University Park Press.)*

Some peptide carriers transport actively and are Na^+-dependent. It should be emphasized that the mechanisms of peptide absorption have not been definitely resolved.

Peptides that enter enterocytes are hydrolyzed by cytoplasmic peptidases to amino acids. These, in turn, diffuse or are moved by carrier-mediated processes from the intracellular compartment, across the basolateral membrane, into the blood. A small percentage of peptides enter the blood intact, which may explain why certain biologically active peptides exert their effects when given orally.

Abnormalities in Protein Assimilation

Pancreatic insufficiency caused by various diseases, including cystic fibrosis and hereditary pancreatitis, may be associated with a decrease or absence of trypsin and lead to poor digestion of protein. Cases of primary proteinase deficiency caused by congenital trypsinogen deficiency have been reported. In those patients, chymotrypsin and carboxypeptidase activities are lacking also, because trypsin cannot be formed to activate the precursors of these pancreatic proteases.

Intestinal malabsorption of amino acids occurs in various hereditary diseases. Knowledge of intestinal transport abnormalities of this type is important, not only for understanding the pathogenesis of certain diseases but also for providing important information regarding the physiological process involved in intestinal transport.

Cystinuria is a disease characterized partly by defective transport of cystine in the proximal renal tubule and the small bowel (Fig. 11-11). Although the intestinal malabsorptive condition is of little or no consequence in the disability produced by cystinuria, the fact that it is limited to the basic amino acids is supportive evidence that specific carrier systems exist for the intestinal uptake of amino acids.

Hartnup disease is a hereditary condition in which the active transport of several neutral amino acids is deficient in both the renal tubules and the small intestine. The intestinal defect contributes to the pathogenesis of this disorder. An interesting finding is that, although neutral amino acids are not absorbed, they readily appear in the blood when their dipeptides are fed to patients. This is compelling evidence that absorption of the dipeptides of certain amino acids is by a completely separate process from the one involved in the transport of free amino acids.

LIPID ASSIMILATION

Dietary lipids are complex organic compounds and include such substances as phospholipids, sterols, hydrocarbons, and waxes that comprise cell walls or membranes of plants and/or animals. Other lipids or related dietary constituents are fat droplets (triglycerides) and fat-soluble vitamins (A, D, E, K). The principles of lipid assimilation will be dealt with through a consideration of triglycerides, phospholipids, and sterols. The propensity of lipids to form ester linkages and the insolubility of lipids in water are important properties to keep in mind in relation to digestion and absorption.

Unlike carbohydrates and proteins, lipids enter epithelial cells by a sequence of chemical and physical events that render water-insoluble molecules capable of being absorbed by passive diffusion. The process depends upon four major events: (1) secretion of bile and various lipases, (2) emulsification, (3) enzymatic hydrolysis of ester linkages, and (4) the solubilization of lipolytic products within bile salt micelles.

Digestion

Fat assimilation begins in the stomach, where food (partially digested by pepsin) is churned into a coarse mixture and released in small portions into the duodenum. Except for short-chain fatty acids, there is no absorption of fat from the stomach. There appears to be a process, controlled through the action of CCK, that slows gastric motility and emptying when fat is in the small intestine. CCK also stimulates the pancreas to secrete lipase and causes contraction of the gallbladder. One function of bile salts released into the duodenum is to perpetuate the emulsification of fat droplets by decreasing the surface tension at the oil-water interface. The emulsification process is important to increasing the surface area of lipids in preparation for their enzymatic hydrolysis.

Enzymes from three sources are involved in the digestion of dietary lipids. These include food-bearing lipases, lingual lipase, and pancreatic lipases.

Enzymes that digest dietary lipids can be found in food per se (for example, acid lipases and phospholipases). These enzymes may function in autodigestion, a process aided by the acid environment of the stomach. Human milk contains a lipase similar in chemical properties to bile salt–stimulated lipase secreted by the pancreas. Known as carboxylic ester hydrolase (CEH), it is active against cholesterol and vitamin A esters. Milk lipase and CEH also hydrolyze glycerol esters of long-chain fatty acids at the physiological pH of the small bowel. A feature that distinguishes these esterases from well-known pancreatic lipase is that the latter has pronounced specificity for the 1 and 3 ester bonds of triglycerides, whereas milk lipase and CEH show no positional specificity. Despite the lack of a clear functional role, it is presumed that milk lipase working in conjunction with CEH is important to the utilization of milk lipids in newborn infants, who have a low intestinal bile salt concentration and absorb glycerol and free fatty acids better than monoglycerides. This presumption is compatible with knowledge that

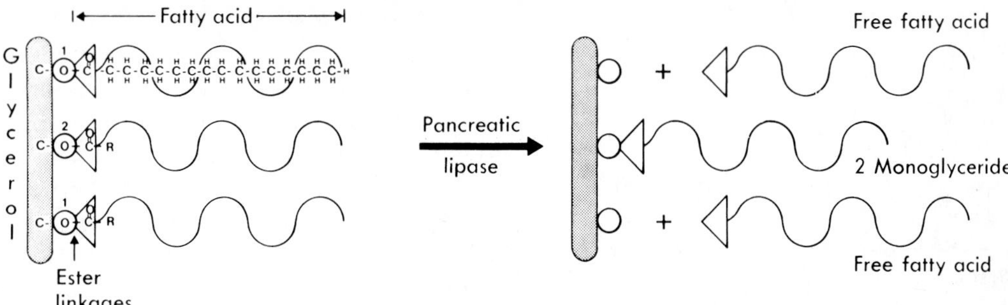

Fig. 11-12. Positional specificity of pancreatic lipase.

milk lipase is stable between pH 3.5 and 9 and is broken down only slowly by pepsin. Thus most of the enzyme would pass through the infant's stomach without denaturation. The fact that it requires bile salts for activation suggests that it is not functional until it reaches the small intestine.

Lipolytic activity in the stomach currently is believed to be caused by a lingual lipase secreted by serous glands of the tongue. Knowledge of lingual lipase has been derived primarily from experimental animals. Indications are that this lipase has a pH optimum between 2.2 and 6 and acts on triglyceride esters. Lingual lipase acts primarily at the outer ester linkages, producing fatty acids and diglycerides. Its proposed function is in the emulsification process, promoting the action of pancreatic lipase.

Pancreatic lipase-colipase, phospholipase A_2, and cholesterol esterase (nonspecific lipase) all function within the intestinal lumen.

Pancreatic lipase, or glycerol-ester lipase, is secreted in an active form rather than as a precursor enzyme. It displays optimum activity at pH 8 and remains active down to pH 3.0. A more acidic pH destroys the enzyme. Although bile salts inhibit its enzymatic activity, this is prevented under physiological circumstances by the combination of lipase with colipase. Colipase, a polypeptide (102 to 107 amino acids) secreted by the pancreas along with lipase in a 1:1 ratio, is secreted as procolipase that is activated when hydrolyzed by trypsin to a peptide containing 96 amino acids. Whereas lipase-colipase complexes are scarce within the duodenum during fasting, the presence of fat stimulates the secretion of these components in large quantities. The inactivation of lipase by bile salts and the prevention or reversal of inactivation by colipase are not understood completely but are theorized to be related to the capacity of bile salts to displace lipase at the oil-water interface, where it must exert its action, and to the obverse capacity of colipase to replace the bile salts at this interface. Once colipase attaches to the oil-water interface, lipase will bind to a specific site on the colipase molecule and consequently carry out its catalytic function, breaking down triglycerides.

Lipase is secreted in large excess and rapidly hydrolyzes triglycerides. The enzyme shows positional specificity. It cleaves the 1 and 3 ester linkages, yielding free fatty acids and 2-monoglycerides. Only small amounts of free glycerol (Fig. 11-12) are produced, reflecting the lack of action against the 2 ester linkages.

Phospholipase A_2 is secreted as a proenzyme and is activated by trypsin much in the same fashion as trypsinogen is converted to active form (that is, through cleavage of several amino acids from the N-terminus). Bile salts

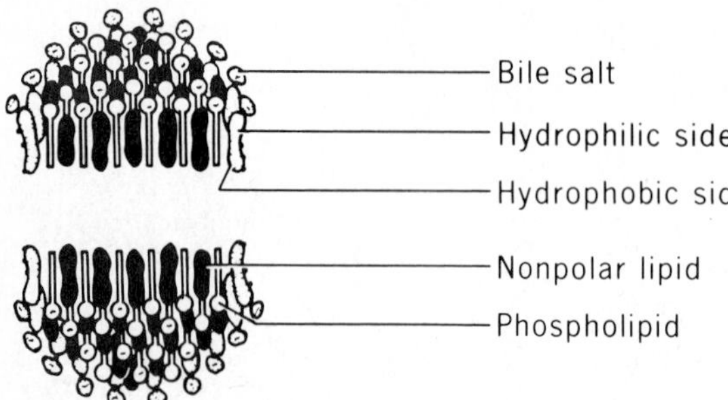

Fig. 11-13. Solubilization of nonpolar lipid by a bile acid–polar lipid micelle. *(Modified from Hoffman AF, French A, and Littman A: Syllabus. Digestion and absorption, Chicago, 1975, American Medical Association).*

and phospholipids form mixed micelles that become substrates for phospholipase A_2. The enzyme has an absolute requirement for bile salts in hydrolyzing dietary phospholipids at the 2 position and producing lysophospholipid and free fatty acids.

Human pancreatic cholesterol esterase hydrolyzes not only cholesterol esters but also the esters of vitamins A, D, and E, as well as those of glycerides. By contrast with pancreatic lipase, cholesterol esterase hydrolyzes all three ester linkages of triglycerides. This capacity accounts for its name, nonspecific esterase. Cholesterol esterase is active against substrates that have been incorporated into bile salt micelles. Activity apparently is dependent on the presence of specific bile salts. The enzyme in humans attacks cholesterol ester in the presence of taurocholate and taurochenodeoxycholate. Esterases from other species may have different bile salt requirements.

Cholesterol esterase is present also in small intestinal epithelial cells. Because the enzyme can catalyze the synthesis of cholesterol esters as well as break them down, it is postulated to function in the formation of chylomicrons.

Absorption of Lipolytic Products

In addition to the functions just mentioned, bile salts perform an important function in the actual absorption of lipolytic products. Sodium glycocholic and taurocholic acids, which are major bile salts, have both hydrophobic and hydrophilic portions. When their concentration in the intestine is raised to a critical level, bile salt monomers form water-soluble aggregates called "micelles." The concentration of bile salt at which molecular aggregation occurs is referred to as the "critical micellar concentration." Conjugated bile salts have a lower critical micellar concentration than do unconjugated ones. Whereas emulsion particles are 2,000 to 50,000 Å in diameter, micelles are about 30 to 100 Å in diameter with a hydrophilic outer surface and a hydrophobic center. The water-insoluble monoglycerides from lipolysis are solubilized within the hydrophobic center of the micelle (Fig. 11-13). In turn, fatty acids, lysophospholipids, cholesterol, and fat-soluble vitamins may be solubilized. A mixed micellar solution is water-clear. Micellar solubilization is important because it enhances the diffusion of poorly soluble dietary lipids through the unstirred aqueous layer overlying the enterocytes.

Two forms of evidence support the participation of micelles in the assimilation of fatty substances. First, mixed micelles (bile salts plus lipids) are found in the intestine. Second, long-chain fatty acids and monoglycerides are absorbed more rapidly from micellar solution than from emulsions.

A major deficiency exists in knowledge related to the process by which lipolytic products dissociate from micelles and enter the enterocytes. Current theories revolve around the importance of the unstirred layer in the intestine as a diffusion barrier that must be confronted.

One possible mechanism of lipid uptake by

enterocytes is the absorption of the entire mixed micelle. This proposed mechanism generally is not accepted, however, because various lipolytic products are absorbed at different rates. Also, because bile salts are absorbed in the ileum, and lipid absorption usually is completed in the midjejunum, it is unlikely that the whole micelle enters the intestinal epithelium. Once absorption takes place, bile salts are transported back to the liver for resecretion. The process of bile secretion, absorption, and return to the liver is referred to as the "enterohepatic circulation."

The most plausible current concept regarding mucosal uptake states that an equilibrium exists between lipids in the micellar phase and in the aqueous phase. Lipids in the aqueous phase may collide with and become incorporated into other micelles or may contact and diffuse through the brush border membrane of enterocytes, shifting the equilibrium between products in the micelle and those in the unstirred layer and causing further release from the micelles. According to this model, absorption of lipolytic products into the enterocyte is determined by the concentration of products in true solution. The latter, in turn, is controlled by the concentration of lipid products in the micelles. Short- and medium-chain fatty acids are not dependent on micelles for uptake because of their higher solubility in and diffusion through the unstirred aqueous layer.

Intracellular Events

Monoglycerides and free fatty acids absorbed by enterocytes are resynthesized into triglycerides by two different pathways: the major one, monoglyceride acylation; and the minor one, phosphatidic acid (Fig. 11-14).

Monoglyceride Acylation Pathway. The monoglyceride acylation pathway involves the synthesis of triglycerides from 2-monoglycerides and coenzyme A (CoA)–activated fatty acids. Acyl-CoA synthetase is the enzyme that acylates fatty acids. The enzymes monoglyceride and diglyceride acyltransferases are responsible for catalyzing the formation of diglycerides and triglycerides respectively. The enzymes involved in this pathway are associated with the smooth endoplasmic reticulum.

An interesting aspect of intracellular triglyceride synthesis is that certain fatty acids are used in preference to others. This occurs despite similar rates of absorption by enterocytes and similar rates of enzymatic CoA activation and glyceride esterification. These observations have been explained by the presence of intracellular fatty acid–binding proteins (FABPs), which have affinities for fatty acids of different chain lengths and varying degrees of saturation. Such proteins apparently exert their influence after absorption occurs and before esterification takes place.

A current theory on how FABPs operate presumes that absorbed fatty acids bind strongly to the apical membrane of enterocytes. Solubilization is brought about when the fatty acids bind specifically with receptors on FABPs. This facilitates the transfer of the free fatty acids from the apical membrane to the smooth endoplasmic reticulum where esterification into diglycerides and triglycerides takes place. This process is particularly effective in the intracellular transfer of long-chain fatty acids. Short- and medium-chain fatty acids, which show less affinity for the cell membrane, are water soluble and are not bound by specific proteins. Instead they leave the cell in free form and enter the blood directly rather than as reesterified triglyceride in chylomicrons.

Phosphatidic Acid Pathway. Triglycerides also can be synthesized from CoA fatty acids and α-glycerophosphate. The latter is formed from phosphorylated glycerol or from the reduction of dihydroxyacetone phosphate

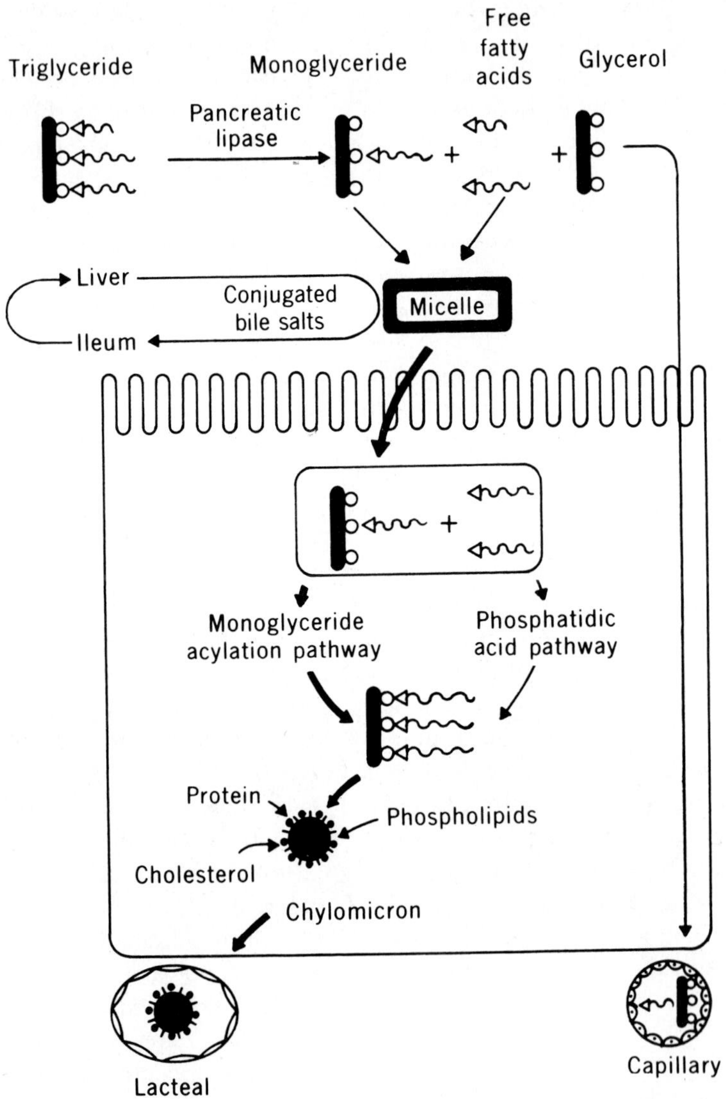

Fig. 11-14. Summary of the digestion and absorption of triglyceride. Monoglycerides and long-chain fatty acids enter the cells after first being incorporated into micelles. Glycerol and short-chain and medium-chain acids, because of their solubility in the aqueous unstirred layer, enter without micelle solubilization.

derived from glycolysis. One mole of α-glycerophosphate acylated with 2 mol of CoA–fatty acids yields phosphatidic acid, which is dephosphorylated to form diglyceride, which, in turn, is acylated to form triglyceride. This minor pathway for triglyceride synthesis in the intestine is termed the "phosphatidic acid pathway."

Phosphatidic acid may be important also in the synthesis of phospholipids such as phosphatidyl choline, ethanolamine, and serine. Alternatively, phospholipids can be derived from acylation of absorbed lysophospholipids by appropriate acyltransferases. The acylation of lysophosphatidyl choline forms phosphatidyl choline, which, along with absorbed phosphatidyl choline, is utilized in the formation of chylomicrons.

Dietary cholesterol is absorbed in free form. However, a major fraction leaves the epithelial cells in chylomicrons as esters of fatty acids. This is indicative of the highly active intracellular reesterification process. The ratio of free to esterified cholesterol in intestinal lymph is influenced by the amount of cholesterol in the diet (low dietary cholesterol favors the cellular exit of greater amounts of free sterol in chylomicrons). In humans the rate of cholesterol absorption decreases as the dietary content increases.

Chylomicrons are lipoprotein particles about 750 to 5000 Å in diameter that are synthesized within enterocytes and exist in the form of an emulsion. Although their chemical composition may vary slightly depending on size, chylomicrons are approximately 80% to 90% triglycerides, 8% to 9% phospholipids, 2% cholesterol, 2% protein, and traces of carbohydrate. It is not evident how triglycerides and esterified cholesterol and fat-soluble vitamins (which form the core) become coated with apoprotein, phospholipid, and free cholesterol (which make up the surface of the chylomicron). Synthesis of both triglyceride and apoprotein occurs in the endoplasmic reticulum, where they form complexes along with phospholipids. This complex, in turn, is transported to the Golgi apparatus, where the protein is glycosylated. The newly formed chylomicrons are secreted into the interstitial space, traverse the basement membrane, and enter the gaps between the endothelial cells comprising the lacteals. Chylomicrons are too large to enter the pores of blood capillaries.

It is evident that apoprotein synthesis by epithelial cells and its incorporation into chylomicrons are essential for fat absorption. Inhibition of protein synthesis causes large amounts of triglyceride to accumulate intracellularly. Several apoproteins (termed A, B, C, and E) have been identified in intestinal lymph. Apoprotein B is similar immunologically to plasma very low–density lipoprotein (VLDL) and low-density lipoprotein (LDL) but chemically and physically shows some uniqueness. It has been suggested that VLDL and LDL in intestinal plasma may represent chylomicrons of varying densities. Generally, however, the role of apoproteins in fat absorption and metabolism is only vaguely understood and remains a current area of active investigation.

Abnormalities in Lipid Assimilation

Impaired lipid assimilation is considered under the general title of malabsorption. In most cases all nutrients are malabsorbed to some extent. However, the definition of the clinical entity is in terms of fat malabsorption because, unlike carbohydrates and proteins, fat is not absorbed in the small intestine but passes through the colon and appears in the feces in a measurable form.

Excessive fat in the stool can be established by extracting fecal samples with organic solvents and determining the total fatty acids present, excluding volatile short-chain acids. Less than 7 g of fecal fatty acid per day is normal. Values above this level suggest malabsorption.

A convenient way to consider fat malabsorption is to take the various steps in assimilation and consider possible derangements. For each derangement there is at least one possible disease:

- Disorders of gastric mixing and intestinal motility do not have any clearcut disease associated with them, although malabsorption may follow the rapid gastric emptying that accompanies partial gastrectomy. Also, rapid intestinal transit has been suggested as the basis for diarrhea in hyperthyroidism.
- Luminal digestion of triglycerides may be deranged by defects in pancreatic enzyme secretion or action. A quantitative defect would be caused by impaired enzyme synthesis and secretion, as occurs with cystic fibrosis (a congenital disease of exocrine glands) or chronic pancreatitis. It should be noted that normal digestion can proceed with as little as 10% to 15% of normal enzyme secretion. A qualitative defect would occur if the conditions for enzyme action were not optimal (as in gastric acid hypersecretion [Zollinger-Ellison syndrome], when the pH of the duodenal contents is lowered and lipase cannot function or may even be denatured).
- Transport from the lumen is a special step in fat absorption and is dependent on a suitable bile acid concentration, which may be low because of a quantitative bile acid deficiency that occurs with an interrupted enterohepatic circulation (for example, ileal resection or dysfunction, or biliary obstruction). There may be a qualitative deficit of the bile acids in a condition known as the "bacterial overgrowth syndrome" (in which stasis in the upper intestine leads to bacterial overgrowth, with deconjugation of bile acids by the bacteria). Free bile acids are absorbed passively in the jejunum because they are largely un-ionized at the duodenal pH. Bile acids need to be ionized to form micelles. Therefore the un-ionized state leads to impairment of fat absorption as well as impaired absorption of cholesterol and fat-soluble vitamins.
- Mucosal cell transport is, of course, necessary for all nutrients; but it is of particular importance in fat absorption, because the absorbed fatty acids or monoglycerides must be reconstituted to triglycerides and then formed into chylomicrons. No disease has been associated with triglyceride synthesis; however, there is a disease of inadequate chylomicron formation, a betalipoproteinemia.
- Lymphatic transport is necessary for the absorption of fat that has been reconstituted to chylomicrons. This step is defective in two rare diseases, congenital lymphagiectasis and Whipple's disease.

Thus by considering the steps in fat absorption it is possible to predict the diseases that can lead to malabsorption. Steatorrhea, which attends malabsorption, can be alleviated to a large degree by diets containing triglycerides of medium- rather than long-chain fatty acids. The explanation for this is that glycerol esters of medium-chain fatty acids are hydrolyzed faster than are ester linkages involving long-chain fatty acids. Medium-chain fatty acids are water soluble and can be absorbed from aqueous solution. Also they are transported directly into portal blood without involvement of chylomicrons.

VITAMINS

Vitamins are organic compounds that cannot be manufactured by the body but are vital for metabolism. They will be considered in this instance, not on the basis of any physiological function, but on the basis of whether they are water soluble or fat soluble (Table 11-3). This feature is emphasized because their solubility characteristic dictates the general mechanism by which vitamins are absorbed.

Water-soluble vitamins are represented by an array of compounds. The principles that apply to the absorption of hexoses and amino acids apply to the absorption of vitamins as well. Strongly ionized or high–molecular weight compounds are absorbed poorly compared with nonionized, low–molecular weight substances.

Relatively little information exists regarding the processes involved in the intestinal uptake of vitamins. Most evidence suggests that passive diffusion is the predominant mechanism. Exceptions to this view exist for thiamine, vitamin C, folic acid, and vitamin B_{12}, for which special transport mechanisms have been reported.

At low luminal concentrations, thiamine (vitamin B_1) can be absorbed in the jejunum of some species, including humans, by a Na^+-dependent, active process, whereas at high concentrations passive diffusion predominates. The presence of a carrier-mediated transport system is suggested by the fact that metabolic inhibitors, thiamine analogues, and the absence of sodium all depress thiamine uptake by enterocytes. Riboflavin (vitamin B_2) is absorbed in the proximal small bowel by facilitated transport. Pyridoxine (vitamin B_6) is absorbed by simple diffusion.

Vitamin C is required in only a few species, including humans. Humans are capable of absorbing it from the intestine by passive processes and also by active transport (an energy-dependent process, requiring Na^+). In rats and hamsters, species that do not require ascorbic acid, uptake of the vitamin occurs only by passive mechanisms.

Table 11-3 Solubility of vitamins

Vitamin	Fat soluble	Water soluble
A	+	
B_1 (thiamine)		+
B_2 (riboflavin)		+
Niacin		+
C (ascorbic acid)		+
D	+	
E	+	
K	+	
Folic acid		+
B_6 (pyridoxine, pyridoxal, pyridoxamine)		+
B_{12}		+
Pantothenic acid		+
Biotin		+

Folic acid has been reported to be transported actively in the duodenum and jejunum of humans and from the entire small intestine of some rodents. A mediated process might be predicted from two facts: folic acid is a strongly electronegative compound (with a molecular weight of 441), and uncouplers of respiration (hence, energy production) interfere with its absorption.

Vitamin B_{12} (cobalamin) absorption requires intrinsic factor, a glycoprotein secreted by the parietal cell of the gastric mucosa. Binding of intrinsic factor to dietary vitamin B_{12} is necessary for attachment to specific receptors located in the brush border of the ileum. Initially cobalamin is released from foods by the action of pepsin. Because of a higher affinity for R proteins (glycoproteins), which are secreted in gastric juice along with intrinsic factor, the vitamin and R proteins form a complex. When the R protein becomes digested in the duodenum, the vitamin then forms a complex with intrinsic factor that is resistant to digestion. The presence of Ca^{++} or Mg^{++} and an alkaline pH is necessary for optimal attachment of the intrinsic factor–B_{12} complex to the receptor, a process that does not require energy. The actual uptake of B_{12} is presumed to be by pinocytosis; however, this point is not clear. Any disease condition that interferes with the production or secretion of intrinsic factor or with the attachment of the intrinsic factor–B_{12} complex to its receptor in the ileum leads to malabsorption of vitamin B_{12}.

The fat-soluble vitamins (A, D, E, and K) depend upon solubilization within bile salt micelles for intestinal absorption. Vitamin A, or retinol, is ingested as β-carotene and absorbed as such. Once in the enterocyte, β-carotene is cleaved intracellularly into two retinol molecules. Esters of dietary vitamin D and E, as noted earlier in this chapter, are digested by cholesterol ester hydrolase before their solubilization in micelles. Dietary vitamin K (K_1) is absorbed in the intestine by an active transport system, while bacterially derived K_2 is taken up passively from the lumen. Except for retinol, which is reesterified, the fat soluble vitamins appear in exocytosed chylomicrons biochemically unaltered by metabolic processes within the enterocyte. The chylomicrons are then extruded into the lymphatics and transported via the thoracic duct into the blood.

SUGGESTED REFERENCES

Ahnen DJ: Nutrient assimilation. In Kelly WN, editor: Textbook of internal medicine, Philadelphia, 1989, JB Lippincott Co.

Alpers DH: Digestion and absorption of carbohydrates and proteins. In Johnson LR, editor: Physiology of the gastrointestinal tract, ed 2, New York, 1987, Raven Press.

Milne MD: Hereditary disorders of intestinal transport. In Smythe DH, editor: Intestinal absorption, New York, 1974, Plenum Publishing Corp.

Rose RC: Intestinal absorption of water-soluble vitamins. In Johnson LR, editor: Physiology of the gastrointestinal tract, New York, 1987, Raven Press.

Shiau Y-F: Lipid digestion and absorption. In Johnson LR, editor: Physiology of the gastrointestinal tract, ed 2, New York, 1987, Raven Press.

Solomon T: Pancreatic exocrine function. In Kelly WN, editor: Textbook of internal medicine, Philadelphia, 1989, JB Lippincott Co.

Wellner D and Meister A: A survey of inborn errors of amino acid metabolism and transport in man, Annu Rev Biochem 50:911-968, 1980.

12 Fluid and Electrolyte Absorption

Gilbert A. Castro

Minerals and water enter the body through the intestine and provide the solutes and solvent water for body fluids. The electrolytes of primary importance include Na^+, K^+, HCO_3^-, Cl^-, Ca^{++}, and Fe^{++}. Each of these ions has one or more mechanisms by which it is transported across the intestinal epithelium. The purpose of this chapter is to consider these mechanisms and their relationship to water absorption and secretion.

BIDIRECTIONAL FLUID FLUX

During a 24-hour period 7 to 10 L of water enter the small intestine (Fig. 12-1). Fluid derived from food and drink as well as salivary, gastric, pancreatic, biliary, and intestinal secretions contribute to this volume. Of the amount entering, only about 600 ml/24-hour period reaches the colon, indicating that most water is absorbed in the small intestine. Because the average daily fecal weight is about 150 g, of which 100 g is water, 500 ml of fluid is absorbed daily from the colon. This volume represents 10% to 25% of the absorptive capacity of the colon, which is capable of absorbing about 4 to 6 L of fluid per day. Malabsorption of solutes and water in the small intestine may result in enough fluid entering the colon to overwhelm its absorptive capacity and cause diarrhea. This, in turn, can precipitate severe electrolyte deficiencies. Although it is possible that ions and water may be added to the feces from colonic mucosa, the major source of water and electrolytes in a diarrheic stool is the small intestine (Fig. 12-1).

It is evident from the foregoing account that several liters of fluid are secreted into the gastrointestinal tract daily and several liters are absorbed. The volume of fluid moving from blood to lumen (secretion) is less than that moving from the lumen to the blood (absorption), resulting in net absorption. Absorption generally results from the passive movement of water across the epithelial membrane in response to osmotic and hydrostatic pressures. Because of these so-called Starling forces, the consequent bulk flow of fluid is analogous to the flow of fluid across capillary walls. In the absence of food, ions are the most important

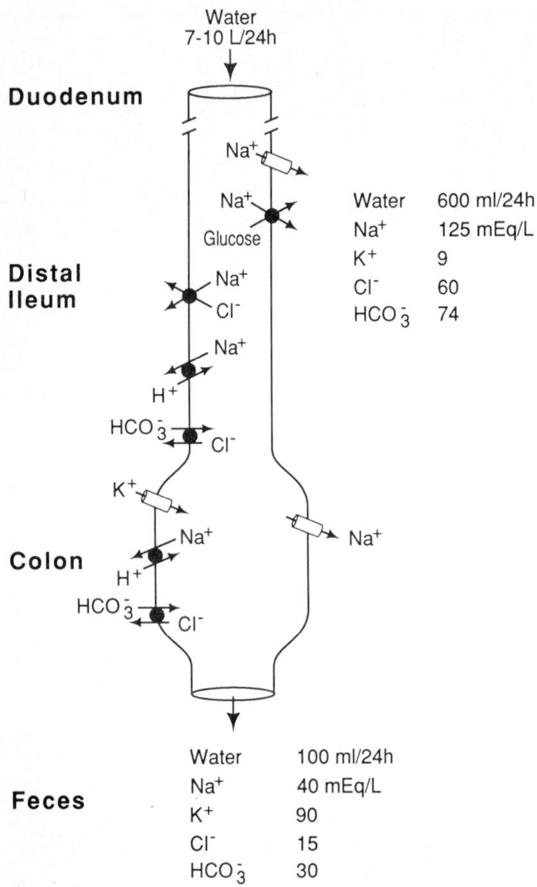

Fig. 12-1. Volume and composition of fluid in the small intestine and colon.

contributors to osmotic pressure in the intestinal lumen. The ionic composition of the luminal contents may vary along the length of the intestine and is different from that in feces. However, luminal fluid generally remains isotonic with plasma because of the relative permeability of the mucosal membrane. The continued production of solutes by colonic bacteria and the relative impermeability of the colonic membrane to water cause stool water to be usually hypertonic, 350 to 400 mOsm/L, to plasma.

IONIC CONTENT OF LUMINAL FLUID

Proceeding from the duodenum to the colon, the Na^+ and Cl^- concentrations in the lumen progressively become lower than the plasma concentrations. In the duodenum, Na^+ is approximately 140 mEq/L, equal to the serum concentration. The major anion is Cl^-. Sodium concentrations decrease in the jejunum and reach about 125 mEq/L in the ileum. The major anions in the ileum are Cl^- and HCO_3^-. Sodium decreases to 35 to 40 mEq/L in the colon, whereas the K^+ concentration increases to 90 mEq/L from 9 mEq/L in the ileum. The major anions in the colon are Cl^- and HCO_3^-.

These values indicate an effective absorption process for Na^+ that becomes increasingly efficient toward the distal portions of the gut. This is caused in part by a decrease in the permeability of the epithelium, preventing the back-diffusion of ions absorbed in the distal portions. Whereas the absorption of Na^+ in the distal gut is effective, the conservation of Cl^- is even more so. Chloride is exchanged for metabolically derived HCO_3^-.

Potassium is absorbed passively by the small intestine as the volume of intestinal contents decreases. The concentration of K^+ remains roughly equal to that in the serum (4 or 5 mEq/L). In the colon, net K^+ secretion occurs. Because of K^+ secretion and the exchange of Cl^- for HCO_3^- in the colon, prolonged diarrhea results in a hypokalemic metabolic acidosis.

TRANSPORT ROUTES AND PROCESSES

Ions move between the gut lumen and the blood by transcellular and paracellular pathways and by several processes. The passive movement of Na^+, both into and out of the lumen, is largely through the lateral spaces. This movement is regulated by the tight junctions or "zonnulae occludens." The rate of this passive component is affected by electro-

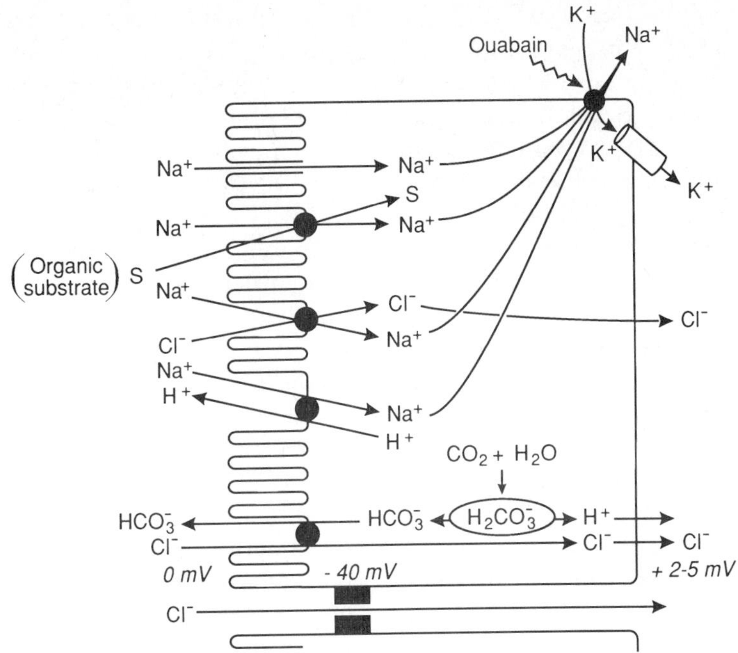

Fig. 12-2. Mechanism of NaCl absorption in the small intestine. Sodium enters passively, following the electrochemical gradient, by cotransport with nutrients such as glucose or amino acids, or by neutral cotransport with Cl^- or in exchange for protons via a countertransport process. Chloride is also absorbed by neutral exchange with HCO_3^-. Sodium exit from the cell is via the energy-dependent Na^+ pump, and Cl^- follows passively. The electrical potential difference across the apical membrane is −40 mV, and across the entire cell is + 3 to 5 mV with reference to the luminal side. Ouabain is an inhibitor of Na^+, K^+-ATPase.

chemical gradients and Starling forces. Normally these forces are small and account for only a small fraction of the net transport. They can, however, be altered under certain conditions, with marked effects.

The tight junction is about twice as permeable to Na^+ and K^+ as it is to Cl^-. Thus electrical potentials can arise across this structure. If, for example, NaCl is moving across the tight junction, the Cl^- will be retarded relative to the Na^+, and the surface toward which the movement is occurring will become positive relative to the other surface. Ions slightly larger than Na^+ and K^+ are much more restricted in their movement.

The pores through which transcellular diffusion takes place are probably larger (7 to 8 Å) in the jejunum than in the ileum (3 to 4 Å). This restricts the passive transport of solutes in distal gut and allows these solutes to exert a more effective osmotic pressure. In turn the reduced permeability makes carrier-mediated transport a more important contributor to net transport out of the lumen.

Na^+-Cl^- Transport

Physiological models describing Na^+ and Cl^- absorption in the small intestine are shown in Fig. 12-2. Sodium is absorbed from the lumen across the apical membrane of epithelial cells by four mechanisms. These include the movement of Na^+ by restricted diffusion through water-filled channels, the cotransport of Na^+ with organic solutes (e.g., glucose and amino acids), the cotransport of Na^+ with Cl^-, and the countertransport of Na^+ in exchange for H^+. Because Na^+-Cl^- cotransport and Na^+-H^+ exchange are electrically neutral processes the driving force for Na^+ to enter the cell is the Na^+ concentration difference between the luminal fluid and the cytoplasm. Sodium movement through pores and Na^+ cotransport with organic solutes are driven both by the concentration difference and the negative electrical potential across the epithelial cell membrane. Thus the entry of Na^+ into the epithelial cell in all four mechanisms is a passive process. There is some question whether the Na^+-Cl^- cotransport system, which has been described in experimental animals, occurs in the human small intestine. Also the contribution of restricted diffusion to overall Na^+ absorption is probably small, relative to other mechanisms.

The Na^+-K^+ pump on the basolateral membranes of the absorbing epithelial cell maintains both the low intracellular Na^+ level and the negative membrane potential. Through this pump the Na^+ that enters by all four mechanisms described above is extruded into the intercellular spaces. The Na^+ pump is the well-known Na^+, K^+-activated ATPase. This enzyme-carrier molecule is activated by intracellular Na^+ and extracellular K^+ to split ATP, releasing energy. In the process, three Na^+ ions are pumped out of the cell for every two K^+ ions pumped in. The pumping out of more Na^+ than K^+ entering creates a potential difference across the basolateral membrane, called an "electrogenic potential." The pump is inhibited by cardiac glycosides (e.g., ouabain). Because Na^+ exit from the epithelial cell is coupled with K^+ entry the intracellular K^+ concentration is much higher than the extracellular concentration. This causes the constant, downhill leakage of K^+ from the interior to exterior by K^+ channels on the basolateral membranes (i.e., the K^+ actively pumped into the cell returns to the exterior through passive leaks).

The epithelial absorption of Cl^- involves, in addition to cotransport with Na^+, countertransport with HCO_3^-. Production of HCO_3^- is by metabolic process taking place within the epithelial cells through the hydration of CO_2 by carbonic anhydrase. Both absorption mechanisms move Cl^- into the epithelial cell against an electrochemical potential difference. The energy for the uphill movement of Cl^- is derived from the downhill movement of Na^+ into the cell or from the downhill movement of HCO_3^- out of the cell and into the lumen.

Because of the transcellular electrical potential difference—the serosal side is positive with reference to the lumen and with reference to the cell interior—Cl^- is driven passively from the cell and into the serosal fluid. Also, luminal Cl^- can move through the paracellular pathway into the serosal solution. The magnitude of this passive absorptive process is governed by the magnitude of the transmural potential difference (PD). That PD is developed through the action of the Na^+-K^+ pump and is influenced by the resistance of the paracellular pathway to ion flow. In the small intestine the relatively leaky epithelium prevents the transmural PD from rising above 2 to 5 mV. In the colon, where the epithelium is less leaky, the PD is about 20 mV. Thus the driving force for Cl^- absorption is greater in the colon.

All regions of the colon absorb Na^+ and Cl^- (Fig. 12-3). However, unlike the small intestine, the cotransport of Na^+ with organic solutes is lacking. Restricted diffusion is the pri-

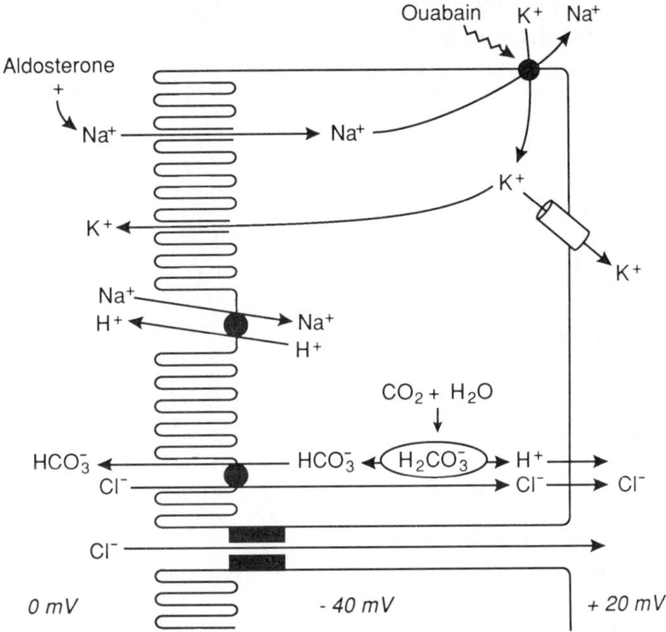

Fig. 12-3. Mechanism of ion absorption in the colon. Na^+ enters passively while Cl^- enters in neutral exchange with HCO_3^-. Net secretion of K^+ occurs.

mary mechanism for colonic Na^+ absorption. This electrogenic process, which increases in activity from oral to aboral regions, is dependent on channels that are under regulation by mineralocorticoids. For example, aldosterone increases the number of Na^+ channels and enhances Na^+ absorption. Sodium in the lumen of the colon also is absorbed through an electroneutral process that includes Cl^- cotransport. This probably involves Na^+-H^+ countertransport coupled with Cl^--HCO_3^- countertransport, as occurs in the small intestine.

A process of NaCl secretion exists in crypt cells of both the small intestine and colon (Fig. 12-4). The mechanism involved is the neutral Na^+-Cl^- cotransport into the epithelial cells at the basolateral membranes. The energy required to drive Cl^- into the cell against an electrochemical potential is derived from the passive movement of Na^+ down its electrochemical gradient. The Na^+ that enters the cell is extruded by the sodium pump. Intracellular Cl^- that attains high levels diffuses across the apical membrane through selective Cl^- channels. These apical channels are relatively inactive under resting conditions but can be opened by an elevation in intracellular, cyclic AMP and/or Ca^{++}. These intracellular messengers can be elevated under physiological conditions, as after a meal, by gastrointestinal hormones (e.g., vasoactive intestinal peptide), neurotransmitters, and paracrine secretions such as prostaglandins. The intracellular messengers also may be elevated to pathological levels by exogenous agents such as bacterial enterotoxins (cholera toxin being the prototype).

The movement of Cl^- from the serosal to

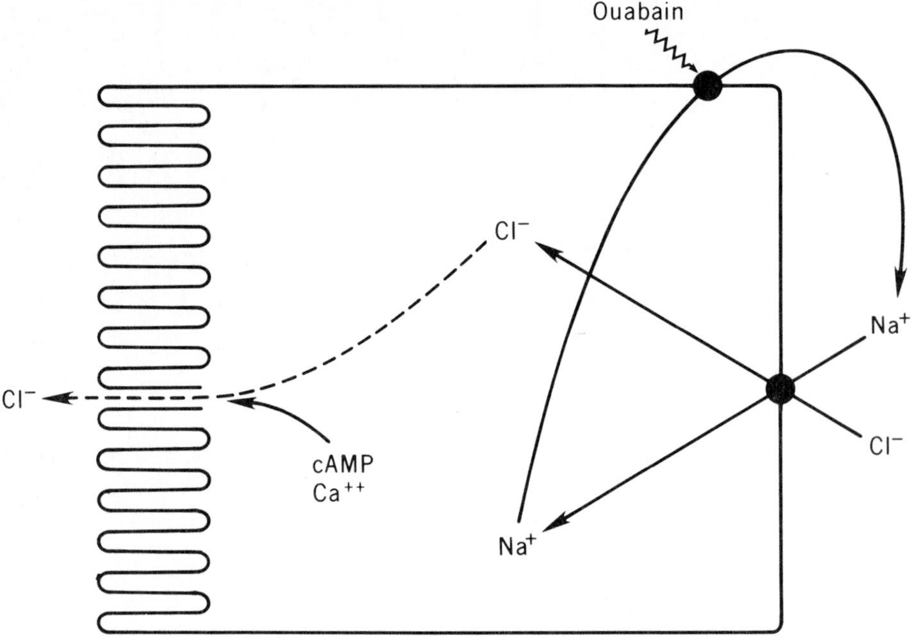

Fig. 12-4. Mechanism of NaCl secretion by the epithelium.

mucosal compartment polarizes the cell electrically, causing the lumen to become negative with reference to the serosa. This electrical potential difference causes Na^+ from the serosal fluid to enter the lumen via the paracellular pathway. Thus NaCl is secreted.

K^+ Transport

Diffusion through paracellular pathways in the small intestine is the primary mechanism by which K^+, derived from the diet or from secretions of the upper GI tract, undergoes net absorption. In the colon (but not in the small intestine) the apical and basolateral membranes are permeable to K^+. Thus, because of the high concentration of intracellular K^+ maintained by the Na^+-K^+ pump, some K^+ leaks passively across the apical membrane of epithelial cells. Factors that elevate intracellular K^+, such as aldosterone-stimulated Na^+ absorption, increase K^+ secretion.

MECHANISM FOR FLUID ABSORPTION AND SECRETION

Water absorption or secretion is always in response to osmotic forces produced by the transport of organic solutes or ions and can be explained in terms of a three-compartment model and local osmotic effects (Fig. 12-5). In the absorbing intestine, solutes are moved from the lumen (first compartment) into and then out of the epithelial cell. This creates a local osmotic gradient, causing water to move from the gut lumen across the cell and into the intercellular space (second compartment). The entrance of water increases the hydrostatic pressure within this space, causing the bulk flow of water and solutes through the basement membrane into capillaries (third compartment). In the nonabsorbing intestine the imbalance of forces across the capillary wall leads to filtration of fluid into the interstitium. However, the capillary filtration rate

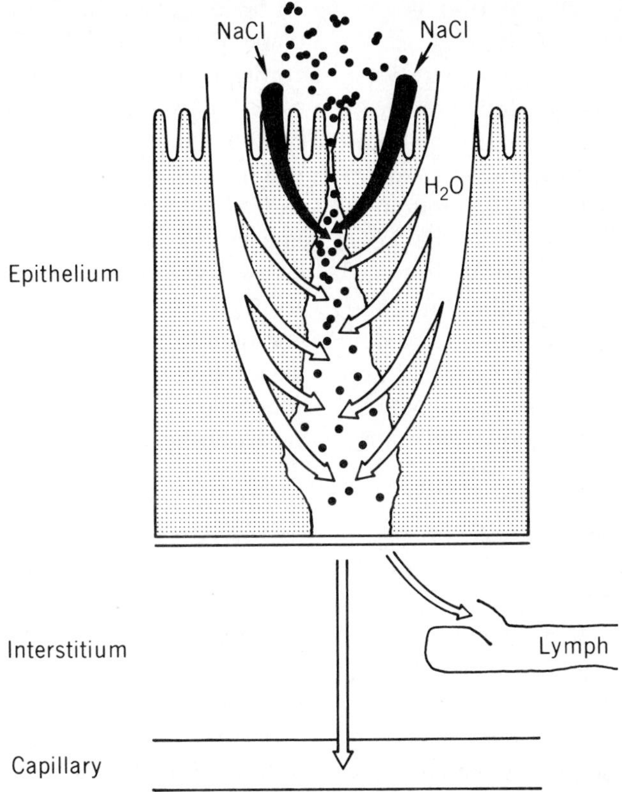

Fig. 12-5. Fluid absorption according to the standing osmotic gradient hypothesis. The sum of hydrostatic and osmotic pressures in the intraepithelial space, interstitium, and capillaries favors fluid absorption. In the nonabsorbing state, fluid filtering from the capillaries would be drained by the lymphatics. The attraction of fluid from the cytosol and interstitium because of high osmotic pressure in the lumen leads to secretion.

is balanced by lymphatic drainage. In the secreting intestine, fluid in the interstitium is attracted osmotically into the lumen.

Osmotic equilibration, and therefore absorption, occur by different means in the duodenum and ileum. The duodenum functions to bring chyme into osmotic equilibrium with plasma. If a hypertonic solution is placed in the duodenum, isotonicity is reached by a rapid flow of water from blood to lumen, increasing the volume of the original solution. More distally, in the small intestine, absorption of solutes creates a gradient for water absorption. Thus the volume is decreased because of both solute and water uptake, and the isotonicity of the luminal solution is maintained during this process. In summary, the sequence of responses to hypertonic contents entering the intestinal lumen is, first, the dilution caused by osmotic attraction of water from the blood and then the movement of fluid from the lumen into the blood secondary to the transport of solutes.

If a hypotonic solution enters the intestine the flux of water from lumen to blood is greater than from blood to lumen, leading to net absorption of fluid. This in turn is followed by the isotonic uptake of fluid.

The gut normally absorbs all electrolytes and water presented to it and, unlike the kidney, does not appear subject to hour-by-hour homeostatic regulation. Nevertheless, some external regulation occurs. The autonomic nervous system has effects on NaCl transport. Adrenergic (α-receptor) or anticholinergic stimuli tend to increase absorption, but cholinergic or antiadrenergic stimuli tend to decrease absorption. Other agents (such as serotonin, dopamine, the endogenous opiates, enkephalins, and endorphins) alter gut transport, usually in the secretory direction. However, the opiates morphine and codeine increase gut absorption.

The ileum has relatively little ability to respond to Na^+ depletion and/or mineralocorticoids. By contrast the large intestine is sensitive to both these assaults which can increase Na^+ absorption and K^+ secretion. Mineralocorticoids can decrease the Na^+ concentration in fecal water from 30 to 2 mEq/L and increase K^+ concentration from 75 to 150 mEq/L. The influence of aldosterone on sodium transport is exerted at two points. There is an increase in Na^+ permeability of the brush border membrane caused by the activation of new sodium channels. Also, aldosterone apparently increases the number of Na^+-pump molecules in the basolateral membrane.

Factors that cause the osmotic retention of water in the gut lumen or stimulate fluid secretion may lead to diarrhea. Saline laxatives such as epsom salts ($MgSO_4$) increase fecal water because of the slow and incomplete absorption of polyvalent ions. Disease states such as disaccharidase deficiency or monosaccharide malabsorption cause osmotic diarrhea. Cl^- secretion that is stimulated by gastrointestinal hormones and neurotransmitters following a meal is a physiological aid to digestion. However, excessive Cl^- secretion, with accompanying fluid secretion, may become pathological in nature. Clinically the ability of the intestine to hypersecrete isotonic fluid is manifested in infections with bacteria such as *Vibrio cholerae* and *Escherichia coli.* The voluminous diarrhea is caused in part by failure of the absorptive mechanism, but largely is caused by the increased volume of secretion. Prostaglandins and VIP stimulate intestinal secretion in amounts comparable to those produced by bacterial enterotoxins. There is the additional suggestion that this secretory effect is mediated through cAMP because VIP, prostaglandin, and cholera toxin stimulate Cl^- secretion in vitro, stimulate adenyl cyclase activity, and raise cAMP levels. The cAMP-stimulated Cl^- secretory mechanism provides a focal point to pursue a physiological explanation of secretory diarrhea.

Ca^{++} ABSORPTION

Absorption of Ca^{++} by the enterocytes is an important component in the regulation of whole body Ca^{++} (Fig. 12-6). The transepithelial movement of the cation occurs against an electrochemical potential. The process, although not entirely known, is localized in the proximal small intestine. Calcium transport occurs in four major steps. First, Ca^{++} absorption involves entry at the brush border membrane. Second, a mechanism must be present to regulate intracellular Ca^{++} levels to prevent altered cell function. Third, vitamin D affects at least one of these steps. Fourth, Ca^{++} exit occurs at the basolateral membrane. In the remainder of this section a scheme compatible with these four points is presented.

Transport of Ca^{++} is initiated by 1,25-dihydroxyvitamin D_3 [1,25-$(OH)_2$-D_3]. This active product is derived from vitamin D_3 (cholecalciferol) formed in the skin by the action of ultraviolet radiation on 7-dehydrocholesterol.

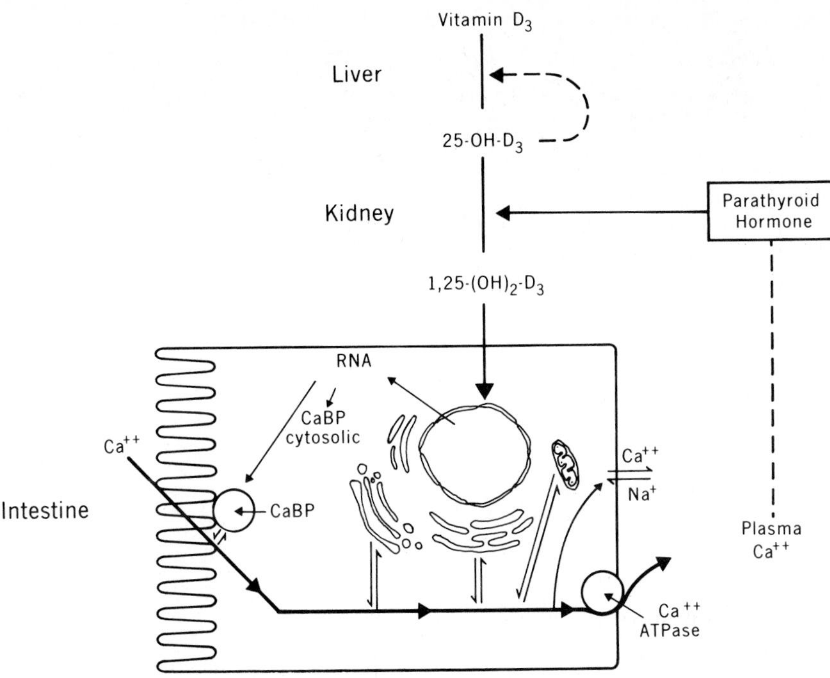

Fig. 12-6. Calcium absorption by an enterocyte within a larger scheme of Ca^{++} homeostasis. Vitamin D_3, 1,25-$(OH)_2$-D_3, stimulates Ca^{++} transport by interacting with nuclear receptors to effect the synthesis of Ca^{++}-binding proteins (CaBP). Ca^{++} enters the cell facilitated by brush border CaBP and exits via two mechanisms. It is speculated that CaBP in the cytosol stimulates Ca^{++}-ATPase. Binding proteins in the Golgi, ER, and possibly mitochondria, prevent a rise in intracellular Ca^{++} during the absorptive process.

Vitamin D_3 is transferred to the liver and converted to 25-OH-D_3. The kidney, through a step regulated by parathyroid hormone, converts 25-OH-D_3 to 1,25-$(OH)_2$-D_3. Enterocytes take up the 1,25-$(OH)_2$-D_3 where it reacts with a receptor molecule in either the nucleus or the cytosol (exact site unknown). The transcription of specific DNA and protein synthesis are mandatory steps in the action of 1,25-$(OH)_2$-D_3 on Ca^{++} transport. The Ca^{++} binding activity of the synthesized protein correlates with Ca^{++} transport. Presumably at least one Ca^{++}-binding protein (CaBP) is inserted into the brush border and facilitates (gates) the entry of Ca^{++} down an electrochemical gradient.

Once inside the cell, CaBPs found in the Golgi apparatus and endoplasmic reticulum minimize the rise in intracellular free Ca^{++}. It has been proposed, but not substantiated, that the mitochondria participate in this "buffering" action. This binding of Ca^{++} by the Golgi apparatus may possibly be a 1,25-$(OH)_2$-D_3–dependent process.

Exit of Ca^{++} at the basolateral membrane is against an electrochemical gradient and involves two mechanisms. The more important mechanism is the Ca^{++}-ATPase, which may be 1,25-$(OH)_2$-D_3 dependent. The other is Na^+,Ca^{++} exchanger, which functions when the Ca^{++}-ATPase is saturated.

Calcium absorption is regulated over the long term by plasma Ca^{++} levels. As intestinal absorption of Ca^{++} rises, plasma Ca^{++} in-

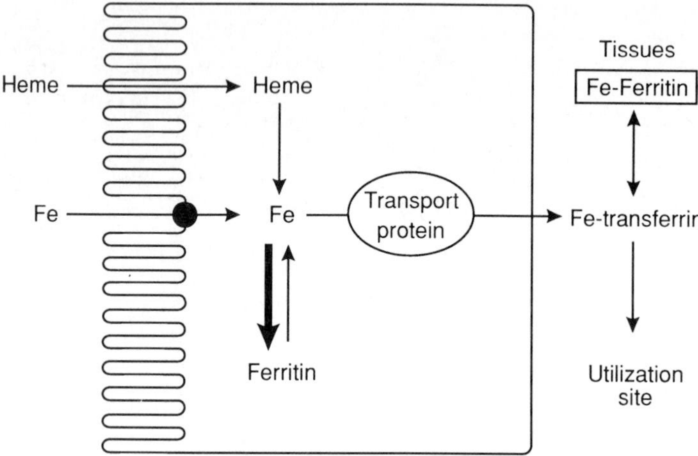

Fig. 12-7. Absorption of iron.

creases; this change inhibits the secretion of parathyroid hormone. In turn, formation of 1,25-$(OH)_2$-D_3 in the kidney is inhibited (Fig. 12-6). A reduction in 1,25-$(OH)_2$-D_3 will eventually cause Ca^{++} absorption to wane, because the synthesis of new CaBP will cease. Although the mechanism of Ca^{++} absorption is not a closed issue, the model depicted in Fig. 12-6 provides a currently popular working hypothesis.

IRON ABSORPTION

Absorption of iron is regulated by total body iron requirements and by the bioavailability of iron. Under physiological conditions, dietary iron is acquired through transport processes in the proximal small intestine. Although the stomach, ileum, and colon have some capacity for iron absorption, this process is most prevalent in the duodenum and jejunum. Normally, because body iron is conserved, absorption of iron by the gut is low compared to the amount ingested.

Heme (derived from meat) is an important dietary source of iron. After it is absorbed intact by enterocytes it loses iron from its porphyrin ring. Heme is absorbed, probably by endocytosis, and digested by lysosomal enzymes to release free iron. In all other chemical forms, iron is absorbed only to the extent to which it can be released from food in ionizable form. Therefore the digestive processes are important in liberating iron. Organic acids such as ascorbic or citric reduce Fe^{+++} to Fe^{++}, which is absorbed more efficiently. Nonheme iron represents the largest fraction of dietary iron, and its absorption will be dealt with in the ensuing discussion.

The cellular mechanism of iron transport has not been completely described. However, a working hypothesis can be synthesized from what is known about the influx of iron across the brush border, its intracellular processing, and its efflux across the basolateral membrane of enterocytes into the circulation (Fig. 12-7).

The initial step in the influx of iron is the binding of iron to a specific receptor on the apical membrane that transports it into the cell. Once inside, some iron is transferred rapidly into the circulation while some is combined intracellularly with a specific protein, apoferritin, to form a complex called "ferritin." A small amount of iron combined with ferritin can be taken up slowly by the body after conversion to free iron. However, most ferritin-bound iron is lost when the epithelium exfoliates. Iron transferred to the blood is transported through the cytosol to the basolateral membrane by a protein that conveys it to the intercellular space. The "transport protein" (intestinal transferrin) is similar to, but not identical with, transferrin. The latter is a β_1-globulin that binds to iron as it exits the enterocyte and transports it in plasma.

The body requirement for iron influences intestinal uptake. Absorption is thought to be regulated at a minimum of two sites. First, it depends on the binding of iron to brush border receptors, whose number is influenced by whole body iron requirements. Second, it is regulated by the ratio of intracellular transport protein to storage protein (ferritin). The formation of ferritin is greatest when the body iron levels are high. Thus iron transfer to the blood is low. The reverse holds during iron deficiency. For example, if iron depletion interferes with body functions such as hemoglobin synthesis, intestinal absorption of iron increases by the formation of more iron receptors on the brush border and by an increase in the intracellular iron transport protein relative to ferritin.

Systemic factors that control or regulate the rate of intestinal absorption of iron remain unknown. However, a feedback system has been proposed that entails both the transport and the storage of iron. Excess iron in the blood is carried to various body tissues, primarily the liver, where it is deposted as ferritin (storage iron), as in the intestinal mucosa. Ferritin-stored iron is in equilibrium with transferrin. During high storage conditions, transferrin in the plasma becomes saturated and can accept no more iron from parenchymal tissue stores or from mucosal cells. Thus iron absorption from the mucosa decreases. The existence of this feedback system and the factors that regulate the cellular mechanism of iron transport in the mucosa remain to be established.

SELECTED REFERENCES

Bronner F, Lipton J, Pansu D, Buckley M, Singh R, and Miller A: Molecular and transport effects of 1,25-dehydroxyvitamin-D_3 in rat duodenum, Fed Proc 41:61-65, 1982.

Conrad ME: Iron absorption. In Johnson LR, editor: Physiology of the gastrointestinal tract, ed 2, New York, 1987, Raven Press.

Dharmsathaphorn K: Intestinal water and electrolyte transport. In Kelly WN, editor: Textbook of internal medicine, Philadelphia, 1989, JB Lippincott Co.

Powell DW: Intestinal water and electrolyte transport. In Johnson LR, editor: Physiology of the gastrointestinal tract, ed 2, New York, 1987, Raven Press.

Schultz SG: Cellular models of epithelial ion transport. In Physiology of membrane disorders, New York, 1986, Plenum Press.

Sellin JH and DeSoigne R: Ion transport in human colon in vitro, Gastroenterology 93:441-448, 1987.

13 The Splanchnic Circulation

Eugene D. Jacobson

The splanchnic organs comprise the part of the digestive tract that is located in the abdomen plus the spleen. Their blood vessels, collectively, are known as the splanchnic circulation. This vasculature constitutes the largest regional circulation that is derived from the aorta. More than a quarter of the output from the left ventricle flows through splanchnic vessels. The major function of the splanchnic circulation is to support the broad range of activities associated with the digestive system—secretion, motility, digestion, absorption, and excretion. In addition, the splanchnic circulation is the storage site for a sizeable blood volume, which can be mobilized during exercise. The splanchnic circulation also is seriously affected by life-threatening, common disorders of the general circulation, such as congestive cardiac failure and hemorrhage, and by local diseases of splanchnic organs, such as cirrhosis of the liver and nonocclusive intestinal ischemia.

GENERAL CONSIDERATIONS

The splanchnic circulation is doubly complex insofar as it serves a variety of organs with different functions and its structural arrangement is intricate. Whereas many of the characteristics of other regional circulations can be related easily to the functions of the single organs they perfuse, those of the splanchnic circulation are far more diverse. Thus the coronary arteries serve one organ that has one main function: the heart is a muscular globe that behaves like a cyclical pump. By contrast, the celiac artery perfuses the liver, spleen, stomach, and pancreas; collectively these organs actively secrete several juices, passively transport solutes and fluids, exhibit motility, store and release blood, and constitute a vast metabolic apparatus for general body and local needs. Consequently it would be difficult to know the cause of a sudden rise in celiac artery blood flow: did it result from increased metabolic activity in the liver, from relaxation of the muscular wall of the stomach, or perhaps from increased pancreatic secretion?

Approximate blood flow values for the major splanchnic vessels of a 70 kg adult human subject with a cardiac output of 6 L/min appear in Fig. 13-1. The diagram also

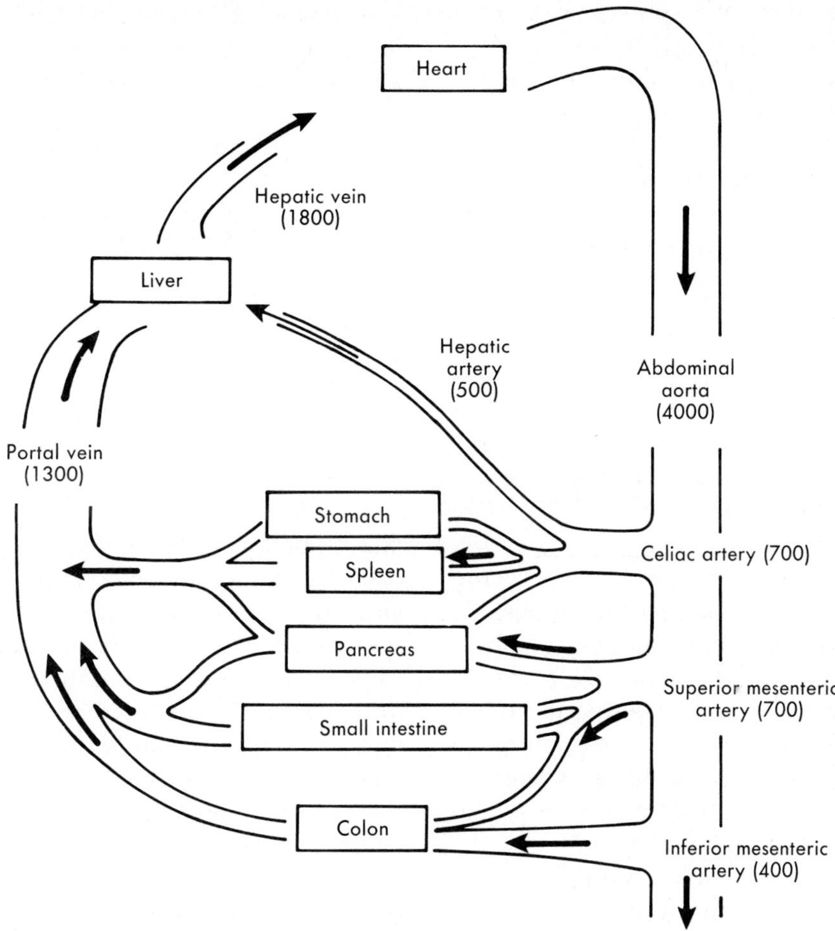

Fig. 13-1. Blood flows and distributions within the major splanchnic vessels of man (milliliters per minute).

shows that the splanchnic circulation is arranged both in parallel and in series. Its three major arteries—the celiac and the superior and inferior mesenterics—form an extensive anastomotic network that is directed to the stomach, small and large bowel, spleen, pancreas, and liver. The hepatic branch of the celiac artery supplies the liver with one-quarter of its blood flow. From the other abdominal viscera, blood drains to the huge portal vein and constitutes the remaining three-fourths of the hepatic inflow. Therefore the liver has a parallel blood supply. The series of splanchnic vessels terminates with the hepatic veins, which drain nearly all splanchnic blood flow back to the inferior vena cava.

CLINICAL TESTS

It is possible to measure splanchnic blood flow using a technique that applies the Fick principle. According to this concept, blood flow through an organ can be measured if the arterial blood carries a measurable marker (such as a dissolved dye), and the marker either is extracted by the organ into its juice or passes into its venous blood. The usual marker is indocyanine green dye. To obtain simultaneous arterial and hepatic venous samples for measurement of the concentration of dye in the blood, a needle is introduced into the brachial artery and a catheter is advanced up the femoral vein and vena cava to be maneuvered into the hepatic vein. Because collection of hepatic bile containing the dye is not easy, an intravenous infusion of the dye is set to flow at a rate equal to that at which the liver extracts the dye from the blood. Because the liver is the only organ extracting the dye, the rate of infusion of dye intravenously is the rate that keeps the concentration of dye constant in the arterial blood.

The splanchnic blood flow can be determined from the following considerations:

1. The amount of dye entering the liver equals the amount leaving the liver.
2. The amount of dye entering the organ equals the arterial dye concentration ($[Dye]_A$) multiplied by the arterial blood flow. The concentration is expressed as grams per milliliter.
3. The amount of dye leaving the liver equals the venous dye concentration ($[Dye]_V$) multiplied by venous blood flow, plus the amount of dye extracted by the liver into the bile.
4. In a steady state, arterial inflow equals venous outflow and either of these is identical to the splanchnic blood flow (expressed as milliliters per minute).
5. The amount of dye extracted by the liver equals the amount being infused intravenously with the pump (Dye infused) and is expressed as grams per minute.
6. The calculation becomes

$$\text{Splanchnic blood flow} = \frac{\text{Dye infused}}{[\text{Dye}]_A - [\text{Dye}]_V}$$

$$= \frac{\text{Grams per minute}}{\text{Grams per milliliter}} = \text{Milliliters per minute}$$

The calculation also requires corrections, because the dye is dissolved only in the plasma, and nearly half of blood is composed of red cells. In adults the resting splanchnic blood flow estimated in this manner is about 25 ml/min/kg body weight. An averaged-sized young American adult male would have an estimated hepatic blood flow approaching 2 L/min. This flow perfuses about 4 kg of splanchnic organ mass, of which the liver is nearly half.

The flow of splanchnic blood is estimated on the basis of the measured rate of indocyanine clearance from the hepatic circulation (Fig. 13-2).

In patients suffering catastrophic occlusion of a major splanchnic artery, it is possible to diagnose and locate the occlusion before surgical bypass or removal of the obstruction by another technique. The radiologist passes a catheter up the aorta from the femoral artery to the vicinity of the occluded vessel and injects a radiopaque solution. Rapid sequential x-ray films reveal failure of the opaque material to flow through the occluded artery. This diagnostic procedure (termed "selective angiography") can indicate which artery should be treated by the surgeon in case of an occlusion or whether an occlusion even exists. It also may be used to remove a clot in a major artery with an intravascular catheter (angioplasty) or to infuse a vasodilator drug into an artery whose blood flow is abnormally low in the absence of a clot.

REGULATORY FACTORS

General Regulators

It has been possible to measure blood flow experimentally and to determine vascular resistance in various gastrointestinal organs and tissues. The gastrointestinal organs generally appear to receive their fair share of blood flow per gram of tissue. The highest tissue flows occur in the mucosa of hollow organs during

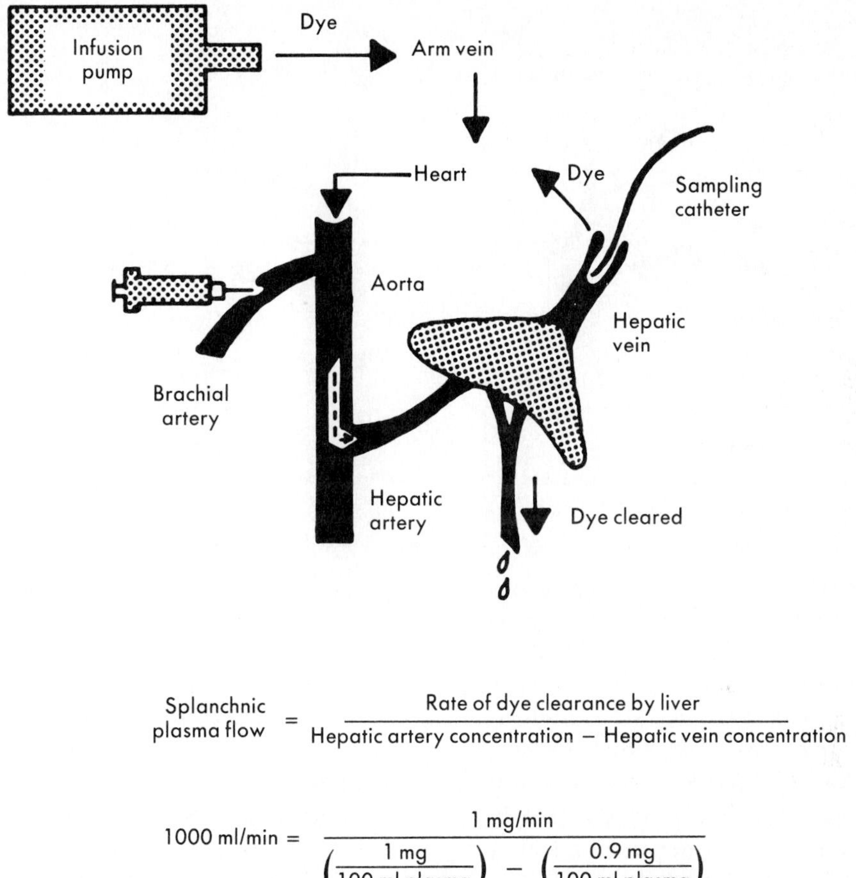

Fig. 13-2. Splanchnic blood flow estimated from hepatic clearance of indocyanine green dye. The dye is infused by a pump into a vein at a rate equal to the rate at which it is cleared from the blood by the liver; hence its systemic arterial concentration is constant. This concentration is measured in samples aspirated from the brachial artery. The hepatic vein concentration is measured in samples withdrawn by the sampling catheter. The calculation of estimated hepatic blood flow for an adult is shown below the diagram. If we assume a hematocrit value of 45, the corrected estimate of splanchnic blood flow will be about 1800 ml/min.

their active state of secretion or absorption (as high as several milliliters of blood flow per gram of tissue). The next highest tissue flow is observed in solid organs, like the pancreas (0.5 ml of flow per gram of tissue). The lowest tissue flow occurs in the muscular outer coat of hollow organs at rest (0.1 ml of flow per gram of tissue).

Each sizable branch of a splanchnic artery coursing over the serosal surface of the stomach or gut gives rise to smaller branches that penetrate the surface and muscular coat of the organ, and eventually enter an extensive submucosal network of small arteries. From this network the mucosal arterioles originate and carry blood to the dense mucosal capillary

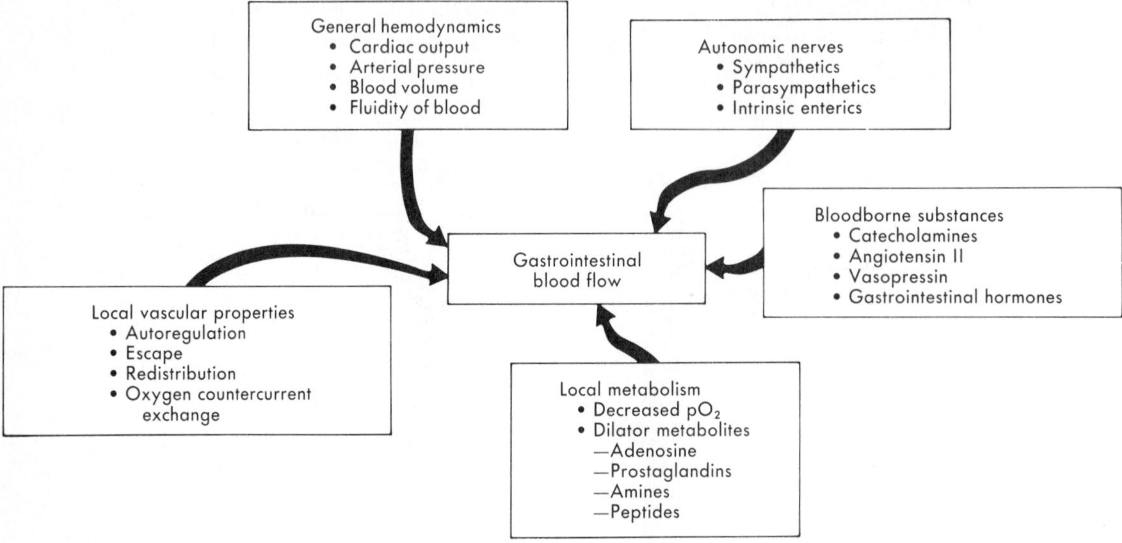

Fig. 13-3. Factors that regulate splanchnic blood flow—including general hemodynamic, autonomic nervous, circulating neurohumoral, local metabolic, and local vascular factors.

beds. The submucosal vascular arrangement guarantees circulatory communication between segments of the gut and leads to great overlap in the distribution of blood by adjacent arterial branches. Such anatomical collateralization helps provide protection against a total loss of blood flow to a segment of gut if its major arterial branch is occluded by a thrombus or embolus. Unfortunately the protection is not enough in the usual patient with intestinal vascular occlusion, because these people are elderly, have generalized arteriosclerosis, and often are in congestive cardiac failure.

In any gastrointestinal organ the circulation is controlled by several factors (Fig. 13-3). General hemodynamic factors include cardiac output, systemic arterial pressure, fluidity of the blood, and blood volume. They reflect the forces that produce an adequate circulation of blood throughout the body. A drastic reduction in any of these factors is reflected rapidly by a fall in gastrointestinal blood flow.

Neural Regulators. The autonomic nervous system is distributed extensively to the splanchnic circulation.

When the *sympathetic* nerves are activated the initial response is contraction of arteriolar smooth muscle with a reduction in cross-sectional area and a rise in resistance to the flow of blood through the organ. As a result there is an initial decrease in blood flow. This response is mediated by the α-adrenergic receptors in the vascular smooth muscle. However, the response is also short-lived and blood flow returns to normal for several reasons:

1. The vascular β-adrenergic receptors also are stimulated, and they cause vasodilation with increased blood flow (through activation of the enzyme that stimulates synthesis of cyclic AMP).
2. The vascular smooth muscle escapes from the constrictive response to the α-adrenergic receptor (discussed on p. 148).

3. When local blood flow is reduced, oxygen tension in the tissue decreases and hypoxia induces vasodilation.
4. Activation of the sympathetic nervous system elsewhere in the body increases venous return to the heart, which elevates the heart rate and stroke volume and increases the flow of blood to all organs including the splanchnic organs.
5. Sympathetic stimulation relaxes the walls of the hollow viscera, thereby reducing mechanical resistance to blood flow through the stomach and gut.

When the *parasympathetic* nerves are stimulated, this affects the splanchnic circulation. In secretory organs such as the gastric mucosa and pancreas, parasympathetic stimulation increases secretion; this evokes an increase in tissue metabolism, with consumption of oxygen and production of CO_2 and various metabolites. The result is vasodilation and an increase in blood flow. In the gut, however, acetylcholine stimulates intestinal smooth muscle contractions, which may generate pressures exceeding 50 mm Hg and impede blood flow through the wall of the organ. Consequently it is not easy to predict the effect of parasympathetic stimulation on blood flow through the bowel. Vasoactive intestinal peptide (VIP), released from intrinsic enteric nerves, is probably responsible for the neurally mediated component of vasodilation during the absorption of lipids from the gut.

Among circulating *neurohumoral* substances are the catecholamines (epinephrine, norepinephrine, dopamine), released from the adrenal medulla, and angiotensin II, formed in response to renin released from the kidney; these constrict the gastrointestinal circulation. As in the case of sympathetic stimulation, their effect is transient. The posterior pituitary hormone vasopressin is also a constrictor agent. Other hormones dilate the gastrointestinal circulation. These include glucagon and CCK (which increase pancreatic and intestinal blood flow) and gastrin (which increases blood flow to the gastric mucosa).

The three sets of regulatory factors just discussed are extrinsic to and distant from the gastrointestinal organs. Closer to the circulation of this system are two other classes of factors—local metabolic and vascular regulators.

When the gastrointestinal parenchymal cells increase their biochemical activities they change their extracellular environment, which is also the chemical environment of the local vascular cells. Increased tissue metabolism resulting from the increased function of the organ causes tissue hypoxia and generates release of many vasodilator metabolites such as CO_2, ions (K^+, Mg^{++}), amines (histamine), polypeptides (bradykinin, VIP), lipids (prostaglandins), and nucleotides (adenosine, cyclic AMP). To a large extent the relationship of tissue metabolism to local blood flow is that of a servomechanism: increased metabolism consumes substrate and produces dilator metabolites that increase blood flow to bring in more substrate; decreased metabolism has the opposite effect.

Local vascular properties of some parts of the splanchnic circulation include autoregulation, escape, redistribution, and the oxygen countercurrent exchanger.

Autoregulation is the ability of a local circulation to maintain a fairly steady blood flow in the face of fluctuating arterial pressures. The decline in blood pressure stimulates local accumulation of histamine. This amine binds to H_1 receptors on the resistance vessels (arterioles), thereby relaxing vascular smooth muscle and increasing mesenteric blood flow to compensate for the decrease in blood pressure. Not all organs in the body exhibit this phenomenon; those showing it include the brain, kidneys, voluntary muscles, heart, intestine, and liver. The protective value of this

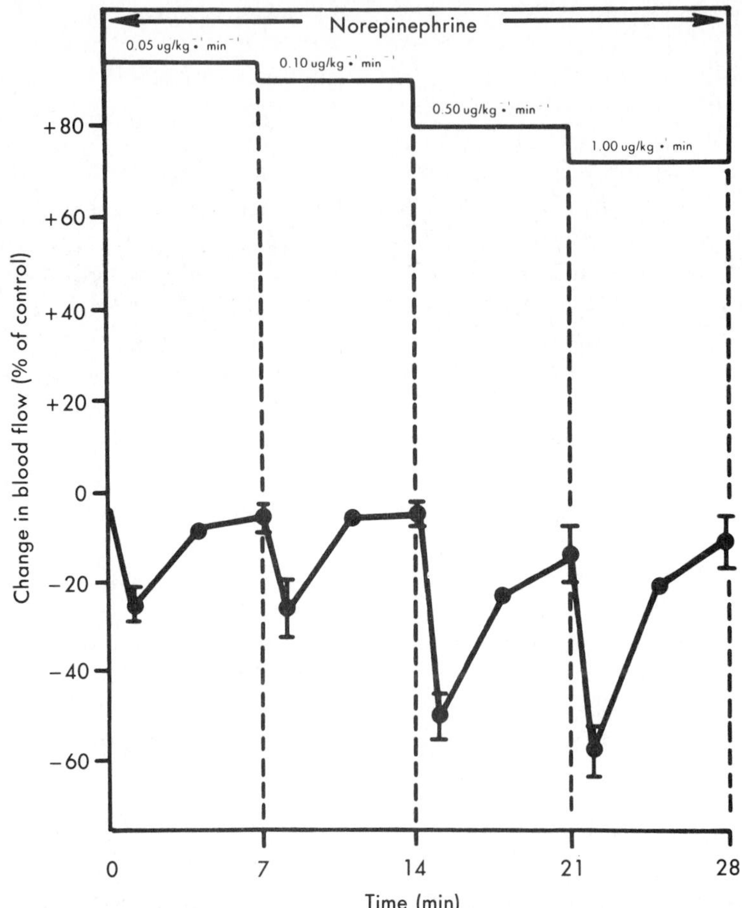

Fig. 13-4. The "escape" phenomenon in the mesenteric circulation. A continuous intraarterial infusion of norepinephrine was set up with progressive increases in dose. With each dose, blood flow decreased initially but quickly returned to the control value despite continued infusion.

property is obvious, because continued functioning of an organ depends on a steady flow of blood. Thus, if the mean systemic arterial pressure is reduced 20 mm Hg by blood loss, flow to the intestines will not be reduced indefinitely. However, a drastic reduction in blood pressure, as in massive hemorrhage, quickly overwhelms autoregulatory protection and lowers blood flow to the gut and liver.

The *escape* phenomenon is similar to autoregulation insofar as local vascular compensations keep blood flow steady in the face of forces trying to decrease flow. During continuous splanchnic sympathetic stimulation and during continuous infusion of catecholamines or angiotensin II there is a transient initial decrease in blood flow to the gut followed by a restoration of flow to normal levels (Fig. 13-4). Increasing doses of a catecholamine are followed by transient reductions in blood flow, despite continuous intraarterial infu-

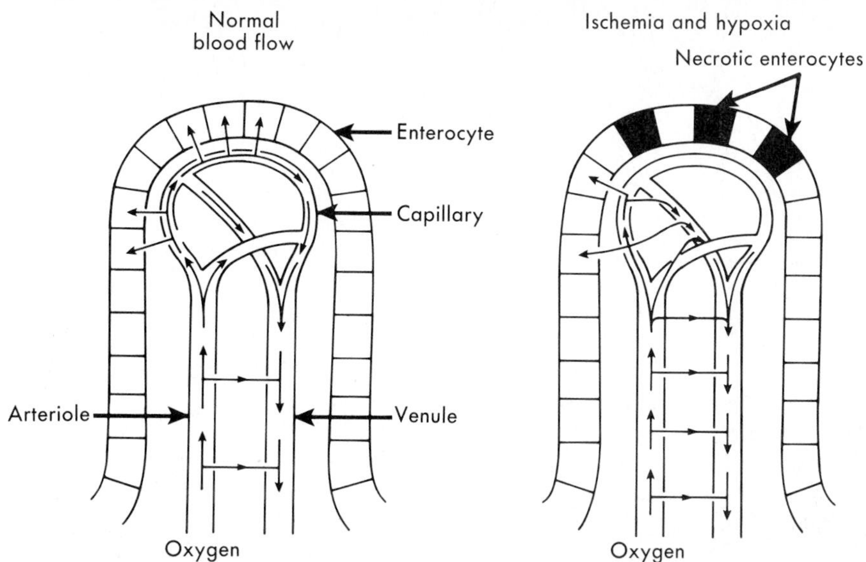

Fig. 13-5. The oxygen countercurrent exchanger. The arterial and venous vessels are very close (20 μm) in the villus shaft. Lipid-soluble oxygen can short-circuit its usual vascular route by escaping the arteriole and passing directly into the venule. Some of this oxygen does not reach the capillaries and cells at the tip of the villus. In pathological states associated with a severe reduction in mesenteric blood flow, the velocity of blood flowing through the villus also is reduced, thereby exaggerating the oxygen exchanger. Ischemic hypoxia at the tip of the villus is intensified, leading to the death of enterocytes.

sion. As with autoregulation the advantage of the escape mechanism to the gut is evident. Escape from sympathetic vasoconstriction appears to be mediated by intrinsic nerves of the gut, which release peptides and purines, such as substance P and adenosine, respectively. These enteric neurotransmitters are released close to arteriolar smooth muscle, where their powerful vasodilator actions overcome the constrictor effects of norepinephrine.

Other vascular peculiarities are not as beneficial to the intestine. Sympathetic nervous stimulation can evoke such a *redistribution* of blood flow within the wall of the gut that mucosal perfusion diminishes and muscular blood flow increases about equally. The result is no change in total organ flow despite mucosal ischemia. The clinical import of this is that angiographic demonstration of an open and apparently normal blood flow through the superior mesenteric artery does not mean necessarily that the mucosa is receiving an adequate blood flow. Thus, in fatal nonocclusive ischemic disease of the gut, a patent mesenteric artery is visualized on x-ray films despite the grossly inadequate flow to the mucosa.

There is an *oxygen countercurrent exchange* mechanism in the villi of the intestinal mucosa (Fig. 13-5). At the base of each villus the inflow and outflow vessels are within 10 to 20 μm of one another, and some oxygen (which is lipid soluble) escapes from the arterialized blood to enter the venule without passing to the capillaries at the villus tip. This creates an oxygen gradient from the base to the tip of the villus, which is detrimental to prolonged cell life at the tip. At normal rates of intestinal blood flow, countercurrent ex-

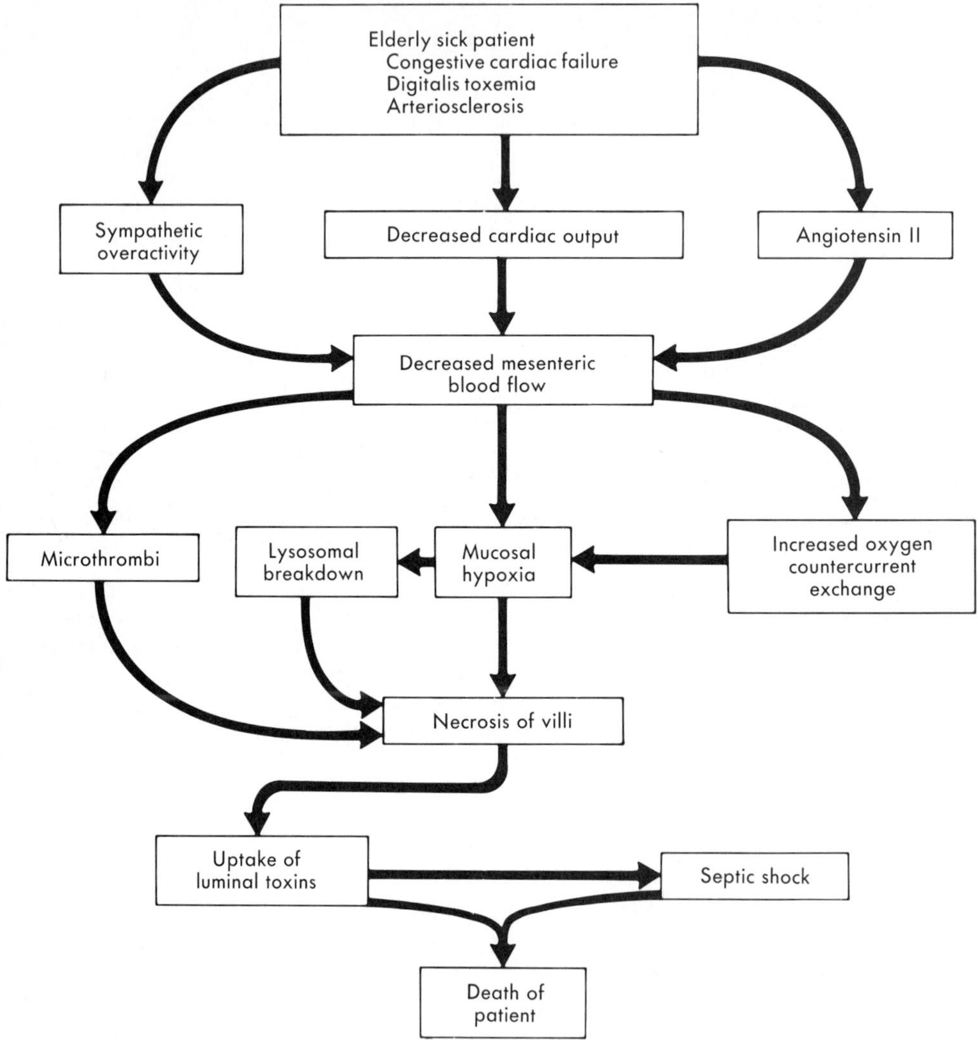

Fig. 13-6. Pathophysiology of fatal nonocclusive ischemic disease of the gut.

change of oxygen is of little consequence; however, when a low flow state develops in the mesenteric circulation the amount of potentially available oxygen bypassing the villus tip becomes considerable. The short-circuiting of oxygen aggravates mucosal hypoxia in ischemic disease of the gut, in which necrosis invariably begins at the tips of the villi.

Regulatory Dysfunction. At this point it is appropriate to apply the preceding information about control of blood flow to a disease of the intestinal circulation. Perhaps as many as 3 of every 100 Americans who die annually are victims of nonocclusive intestinal ischemia. In its severe form the disease is nearly always fatal. The pathophysiological development of this disease is diagrammed in Fig. 13-6.

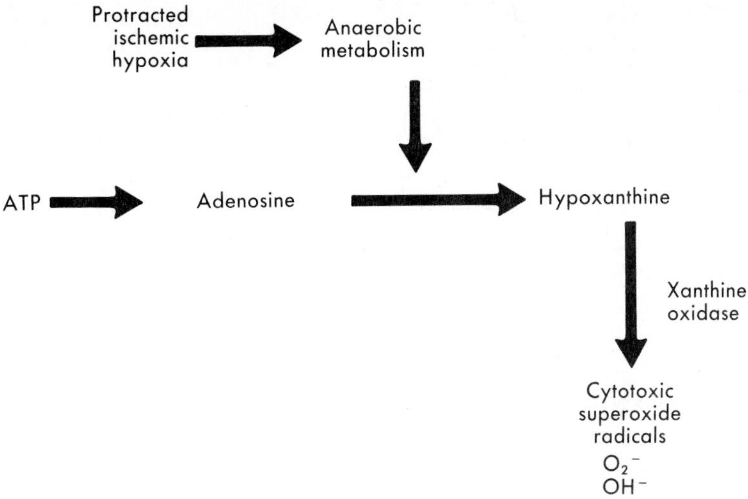

Fig. 13-7. Hypoxic metabolism generates cytotoxic substances. It has been possible to alleviate the damaging effects of ischemia by blocking the action of xanthine oxidase with allopurinol.

The typical patient is elderly, suffering from congestive cardiac failure, and being treated with a cardiac glycoside (digitalis). One day, for no apparent reason, severe and constant abdominal pain develops. When seen by a physician the patient is in circulatory shock (systemic arterial pressure and cardiac output seriously diminished).

Arterial hypotension evokes generalized sympathetic nervous system activation and catecholamine release through carotid, aortic, and pancreatic baroreceptor and chemoreceptor mechanisms. Analogous mechanisms in the kidneys and brain trigger release of angiotensin II and vasopressin, respectively. The declining blood pressure and circulating vasoconstrictors cause small blood vessels to collapse as their critical closing pressures are reached.

The decreased cardiac output is reflected in decreased intestinal perfusion. As the velocity of flowing blood declines the viscosity increases. Furthermore, with a slowing of blood flow through the gut, blood stagnates and microscopic thrombi develop in a disseminated fashion.

Along with the net effect of sympathetic stimulation, release of many circulating vasoconstrictor agents, collapse of splanchnic small vessels, elevated viscosity of blood, and formation of microthrombi, there is an increase in the resistance to blood flow through the gut. In the face of a lower arterial pressure and a lower cardiac output the increased mesenteric vascular resistance means additional reductions in the flow of blood to the intestine. Compounding the ischemic problem are the adverse vascular phenomena—redistribution and the countercurrent exchanger for oxygen—that take oxygen from the mucosal tissue at the tips of the villi. Hypoxic metabolism causes degradation of adenosine into hypoxanthine, which in turn is converted into cytotoxic superoxide radicals (Fig. 13-7). The radicals oxidize the lipids of cell membranes, thereby changing the permeability of cells irreversibly and destroying active transport at the plasma membrane. Cells so damaged can no longer maintain a normal intracellular composition, and they perish. The result is a wide-spread necrosis of the mucosa, beginning at the tips of the villi and burrowing into the mucosa and deeper layers of the gut wall. A main function of the gut is lost rapidly; it no longer serves as a barrier to the absorption of its toxic contents. Many substances are absorbed across the dying inner lining of the gut and pass into the dying circulation. These include bacteria, their exotoxins and endotoxins, myocardial depressant factors, breakdown products of necrotic cells (structural proteins, polypeptides), lysosomal proteolytic enzymes (hydrolases, cathepsins), mast cell products (histamine, 5-hydroxytryptamine), hemoglobin, and electrolytes. The entry of this biological junk into the circulation produces a profound toxemia. Normal body defenses are impaired; the heart is failing; the peripheral circulation is in a state of shock; the abdominal reticuloendothelial system is ischemic; the barrier function of the gut is lost. Then the patient dies.

Regulation of Blood Flow to Specific Organs

Stomach. The circulation of the stomach has been related to its secretory function. When gastric secretion is increased by secretagogues (histamine, gastrin, acetylcholine), gastric mucosal blood flow also increases, and about proprotionally, as seen in Fig. 13-8. When gastric secretion is decreased by secretory inhibitors (catecholamines, vasopressin, prostaglandin E_1, atropine, secretin), mucosal blood flow also decreases as shown in the same figure.

The action of these agents on the circulation of the stomach is twofold. First, by altering secretion, and therefore metabolism, the secretagogue or inhibitor will alter blood flow indirectly by increasing or decreasing, respectively, the release of vasodilator metabolites (cyclic AMP, carbon dioxide). Second, some secretagogues (histamine, acetylcholine) also directly dilate, and some inhibitors (norepinephrine, vasopressin) also directly constrict, the gastric blood vessels. This means, for example, that histamine increases blood flow to the stomach, both because it increases secretion and mucosal metabolism and because it relaxes gastric arteriolar smooth muscle. Conversely, one kind of secretory inhibitor (such as prostaglandin E_1) decreases gastric mucosal blood flow because it inhibits secretion and metabolism, whereas another inhibitor (vasopressin) decreases blood flow because of both its antisecretory and its direct vasoconstrictor properties. Thus, the two major regulatory mechanisms of gastric mucosal blood flow are the rate of gastric secretion (and metabolism) and the constrictor or dilator properties of circulating agents. The role of the autonomic nerves, also, cannot be overlooked. However, the vagi drive secretion (directly and through the release of gastrin) and the splanchnic sympathetic nerves inhibit it. Neural effects therefore infuence gastric mucosal blood flow mainly indirectly and perhaps directly. Hormones like gastrin, secretin, and adrenocorticosteroids appear to act on blood flow primarily through their effects on secretion and mucosal metabolism.

There are two locations in the gastric microcirculation where alterations in smooth muscle tone will change blood flow to the mucosal lining of the stomach. The first location is in the submucosa, where a plexus of reactive vessels exist through which blood flows en route to the mucosa. Vasoconstrictive interventions, such as sympathetic nerve stimulation, act on submucosal arterioles to regulate the flow of blood to the mucosa. Inside the mucosa, arterioles are exposed to the chemical environment of an actively metabolizing tissue, where changes in Po_2 and the concentration of dilator metabolites affect arteriolar tone and, hence, blood flow. At peak secretory rates, over 90% of the entire gastric blood flow perfuses the mucosa.

The question of a relationship between the

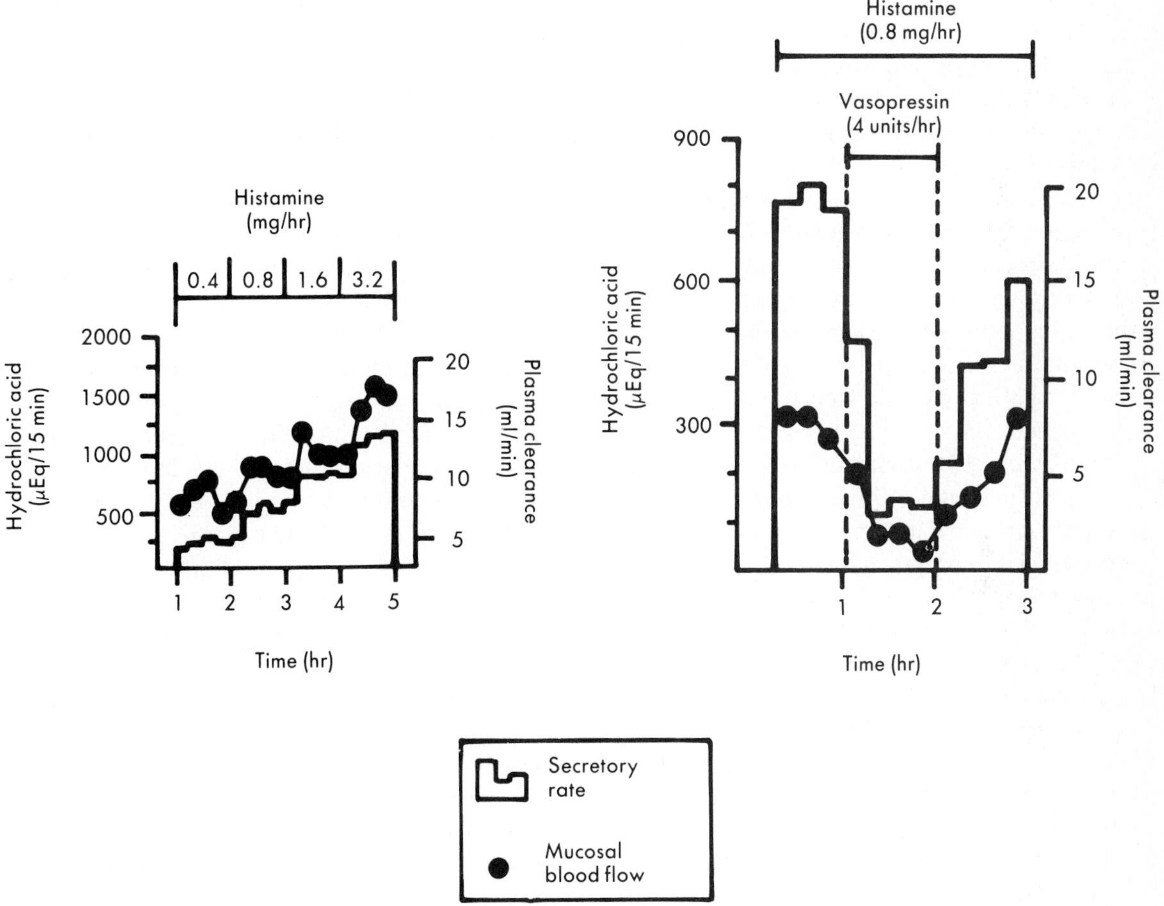

Fig. 13-8. Relationship between gastric secretion and gastric mucosal blood flow. The secretory rate in the stomach is represented graphically by the *bars,* and blood flow (determined from the clearance of aminopyrine from the plasma) by the connected line of *solid circles.* Histamine increases both secretion and mucosal blood flow in a dose-dependent fashion. Vasopressin inhibits both secretion and mucosal blood flow.

mucosal circulation and peptic ulcer disease is intriguing. On the one hand, mucosal ulcerations are provoked by the action of hydrochloric acid and pepsin on a mucosal lining whose resistance to damage has been lowered; an inadequate circulation contributes directly to lowering mucosal resistance. However, experimental findings indicate that mucosal circulatory insufficiency follows, rather than precedes, the events causing ulceration (for example, topical damage with lipid-soluble agents such as aspirin). Furthermore, an acidic juice containing pepsin is necessary for ulcer formation. Chemicals causing ulcers include those that increase (histamine) and those that decrease (vasopressin) both blood flow and secretion. Finally, ligation of 90% of the blood supply to the stomach does not induce ulcers.

Pancreas. The pancreatic circulation, like that of the stomach, is linked loosely to secretion. This means that increased secretion (and metabolism) prompts increased blood flow to the pancreas while decreased secretion is accompanied by decreased blood flow. In addition, the direct actions of powerful circulating vasodilators and neural transmitters must be remembered. Pancreatic secretion, metabolism, and blood flow are enhanced by secretin, CCK, and parasympathetic stimulation.

The effect of eating a meal on pancreatic blood flow is positive. The cardiac output increases, and blood flow is augmented to all organs. Eating activates the vagi, which stimulate gastric acid secretion and emptying of acid and food into the duodenum. Acid and food in the duodenum cause mucosal release of the hormones secretin and CCK. Acetylcholine (released by the vagi and intrinsic pancreatic nerves), secretin, and CCK stimulate pancreatic secretion and metabolism, causing local release of dilator metabolites. Acetylcholine and CCK are also direct vasodilators.

Nerves that release the vasodilator substance VIP occur in pancreatic tissue. The main vasoconstrictors influencing pancreatic blood vessels are catecholamines, which are released by splanchnic sympathetic nerves, and which subsequently bind to α-adrenoceptors on the smooth muscle cells of pancreatic arterioles.

Intestine. Intestinal blood flow comprises more than half the splanchnic flow. The process of seeing, smelling, and tasting food causes an increased cardiac output and increased intestinal blood flow. Beyond this, eating and swallowing the food further stimulate intestinal blood flow and prolong the duration of vasodilation for 3 hours or longer. These effects of feeding are mediated by the conscious and involuntary brain through the vagus nerves, through effects of polypeptide hormones that are released during a meal, and through stimulation of local metabolism and local nerves in the gut.

When food is presented to the gut, blood flow is increased. For example, glucose in the intestine evokes mesenteric vasodilation. During exercise, blood flow to the gut is reduced despite increases in the cardiac output, probably secondary to intense sympathetic adrenergic stimulation.

Visceral smooth muscle in the wall of the gut contracts and relaxes in a coordinated manner, which is referred to as "intestinal motility." These motions serve to propel luminal solutions down the length of the gut, to mix solutions of nutrients and digestive enzymes, and to expose more surface area of the mucosa for absorption of digestion products. These movements reflect increased metabolism of the smooth muscle and lead to an increase in blood flow so long as the tension in the wall does not reach high pressures. However, when the pressure in the lumen of the gut exceeds 25 mm Hg, which may occur with single, intense contractions, there is a mechanical impediment to tissue perfusion, and blood flow will decrease, at least transiently.

An overwhelming disease state that affects the intestinal circulation is shock. As indicated previously in the discussion of nonocclusive intestinal ischemia (pp. 150–152), the circulation of the gut can be a prime target in some shock states and its severe impairment may lead to rapid death. The venous side of the splanchnic circulation is a great reservoir of blood and normally may contain one-fifth of the total blood volume. In some shock states the splanchnic venous capacitance becomes a vast pool of stagnating blood, unable to move its badly needed contents to the rest of the circulation.

Spleen. A major function of the spleen is to serve as a temporary site for the storage of blood, which can be mobilized to meet the needs of the rest of the body. The spleen contains two functionally distinct vascular compartments. The larger compartment consists of the usual array of arteries, microcirculatory vessels, and veins, through which blood either flows or is in temporary storage. More than three-fourths of the splenic blood is in this compartment, and the blood has a hematocrit of about 40%. The lesser vascular compartment of the spleen is located in the red pulp, where the venules are able to trap red blood cells selectively. Blood in this compartment has a hematocrit of 70%.

In response to abrupt hemorrhage, systemic arterial blood pressure declines, and the hypotension triggers central baroreceptor activation of the sympathetic nervous system and release of catecholamines, angiotensin II, and vasopressin into the circulation. These vasoactive intermediaries take quick effect on the spleen, causing constriction of its venular smooth muscle with expulsion of three-fourths of its blood volume. As noted above, splenic blood is rich in red blood cells. These valuable commodities are martialled centrally to offset the cytotoxic effects of hemorrhagic hypoxia on such sensitive organs as the brain and the heart. If the level of hemorrhage is not overwhelming the response from storage sites in the spleen, liver, and voluntary muscle will provide adequate compensation for the initial blood loss. Under these circumstances, moderate hemorrhage may not cause any decrease in blood flow to the kidneys and gut. However, in a splenectomized subject, moderate hemorrhage does reduce renal and mesenteric blood flows as the body tries to sequester blood flow centrally to protect the heart and brain. Thus the circulatory response of the spleen to hemorrhage represents the first line of defense of the body against blood loss.

Liver. The blood supply to the liver is unusual in that three-fourths of the inflow is carried by a very large vein, with the remainder being delivered by a sizeable artery. The blood flowing out of the liver courses through another set of veins. Furthermore the blood that is delivered to the gut passes subsequently to the liver. Therefore, pathological events involving any of these four vessels will threaten the adequacy of blood flow through the liver. Some common examples of such disturbances, which are depicted in Fig. 13-9, include the following;

1. Congestive cardiac failure—the heart is unable to pump blood efficiently, resulting in partial obstruction to the flow of blood out of the liver and elevation of hepatic venous pressure.
2. Hemorrhage—systemic arterial pressure and cardiac output decline and activate the sympathetic nerves to the hepatic artery, which is constricted and experiences a decrease in its blood flow.
3. Cirrhosis of the liver—intrahepatic scarring, following the loss of cells in this toxic liver disease, produces obstruction to the flow of blood, with an increase in portal venous pressure.

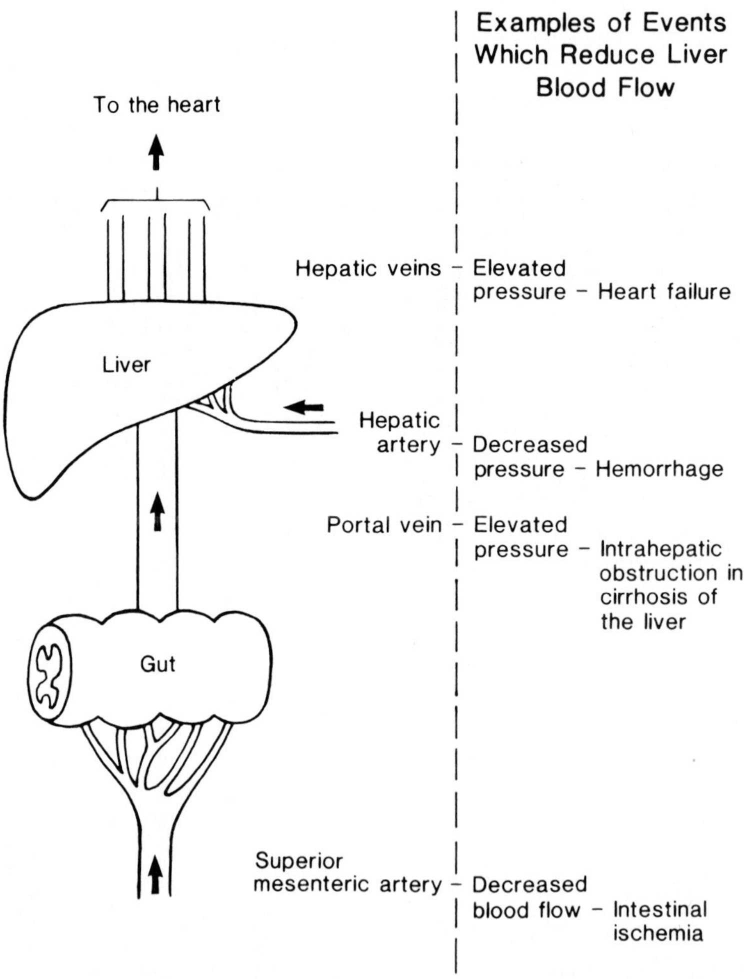

Fig. 13-9. Blood flow through the liver may be reduced by disorders that affect either of its two inflow vessels, its outflow vessels, or the blood flow to the gut. Listed beside each of the four sets of vessels is a major finding in the vessel with a common disease that would be marked by that finding.

4. Intestinal ischemia—extreme vasoconstriction of the superior mesenteric artery reduces blood flow to the gut and also, therefore, to the liver.

The hepatic artery provides one-fourth of the blood supply to the liver. Mean pressure in the main artery is about 100 mm Hg. As the artery branches within the substance of the liver into a myriad of even smaller vessels, pressure falls precipitously, until the arterioles empty their blood into the sinusoids of the liver, where pressure is less than 10 mm Hg. Portal venous blood pressure is 10 to 15 mm Hg in the main vein, and its intrahepatic branches also empty their blood into the sinusoids. Exchange of nutrients from blood to cells, and of metabolites in the reverse direction, occurs across the thin walls of the sinusoids.

Total blood flow to the liver from both the portal vein and hepatic artery amounts to 1 ml/min/g of hepatic tissue. In a healthy adult male this flow comprises about one-fourth of the cardiac output. After ingestion of a meal there is a considerable increase in blood flow to the stomach and gut. The result is an increase in blood flow to the liver through the portal vein.

There are several regulators of blood flow to the liver. Splanchnic sympathetic nerves to the circulation of the liver release norepinephrine, which contracts both venous and arterial smooth muscle. One result is the expulsion of stored blood from the hepatic venules to augment the venous return to the heart. Other effects include a decrease in hepatic artery blood flow and an increase in portal vein pressure. The overall effect is a decline in liver blood flow. These events would occur with exercise or hemorrhage.

The peptide hormones involved in digestive processes (gastrin, secretin, CCK, and glucagon) are released from the gastrointestinal mucosae into the portal circulation. Within the liver these circulating agents relax presinusoidal vascular smooth muscle, thereby enhancing the perfusion of the liver with blood and oxygen. The timing of this vasodilation, which maximizes the provision of chemical energy to the liver at its work peak, is more than fortuitous.

There is also a relationship between portal venous and hepatic arterial blood flows. When portal inflow is reduced, vasodilation of the hepatic artery occurs and more arterial blood flows into the liver. The latter flow is richer in oxygen and compensates to prevent hypoxia of the organ.

THE INTERSTITIAL SPACE

The interstitium of the gut receives vast quantities of water and solutes that have diffused from intestinal capillaries or have been absorbed from the intestinal lumen. The absorbed solutions include about 2 L of digested food and drink plus another 5 L of solutions secreted by the stomach, pancreas, liver, and gut. Nevertheless, most of the material that reaches the interstitium is water, which has been filtered across intestinal capillaries.

The walls of the intestinal capillaries contain special fenestrations that permit ready penetration of water and small solutes from the plasma of the capillaries into the interstitium. In addition, there is a much greater density of capillaries per gram of gut tissue than is found in many other organs of the body. Hence the surface area for diffusion of the ultrafiltrate of plasma is enormous. The main driving force pushing plasma into the interstitium is the difference between capillary blood pressure and interstitial space pressure at the arteriolar end of the capillary. The fenestrations are not sufficiently large to permit macromolecular diffusion, however. As a result of the semipermeable nature of the capillary wall, an osmotic gradient is maintained that returns most of the ultrafiltrate to the venular end of the capillary, thereby preventing the accumulation of excess fluid in the interstitium. Lymphatics also drain fluid from the interstitium back to the general circulation.

Absorbed small molecules from the digestion of food, ions, and water diffuse from or actively are transported from the lumen of the gut, across the epithelium, and into the interstitium. Most of the water and much of the ionic solute diffuses from the lumen through the spaces between epithelial cells to reach the interstitium. Actively transported solutes, accompanied by fluid, cross the apical cell boundary in order to leave the intestinal lumen.

Other absorbed materials fail to penetrate the capillary wall. Instead, such materials diffuse through the fluid channels of the interstitium lying between collagen fibrils. These substances travel a distance of 50 μm before reaching the lymphatic vessels of the intestinal mucosa. In addition to the absorbed materials that reach the lymphatics, there is another source of interstitial small molecules, ions, and water—the substances that have been filtered out of the proximal ends of the vascular capillaries, where the force of the blood pressure exceeds the opposing force exerted by the osmotic pressure of the plasma. Altogether the solutes and fluid accumulating in the interstitium generate a small pressure differential sufficient to initiate a flow of lymph from the gut. At rest the rate of flow is approximately 0.095 ml/min/100 g of intestinal tissue, or 0.1% of the blood flow through the same tissue.

The rate of lymph flow is increased at mealtimes when intestinal absorption is stimulated and blood flow to the gut is increased. The fluid in the lymph, like that of the interstitium, is composed of an ultrafiltrate of plasma to which has been added some of the intestinal absorbate and molecules derived from neural cells (such as VIP) as well as certain enzymes and immunoglobulins.

At mealtimes the increased movement of fluid from the intestinal lumen and the capillaries increases interstitial pressure, thereby forcing more fluid into the lymphatics and increasing the flow of lymph. When the gut is absorbing at high rates as much as 20% of the absorbate is transported by intestinal lymphatics rather than by the vascular capillaries.

Although lymphatics transport many materials that are conveyed by the vascular capillaries, there is one category of solutes that moves preferentially by the lymph—the dietary fats. During intestinal absorption of dietary fats, aggregates of triglycerides containing long-chain fatty acids, cholesterol, and phospholipids are formed in the enterocytes. These conglomerates of mixed lipids are called "chylomicrons." Chylomicrons, which exist in emulsion form, emerge from the enterocyte through a pinocytotic process. The lipids enter the interstitial space of the interstitial villi and diffuse through liquid channels to reach the lymphatic vessel in the core of each villus (lacteal). Entry of aggregates of large–molecular weight lipids and lipoproteins into lacteals appears to involve both vesicular passage across the lymphatic endothelium and diffusion of chylomicrons through gaps in the endothelial membranes.

The mesenteric lymphatics convey solvent and solutes to the thoracic duct. Lymph then flows through the latter vessel to the subclavian vein.

SPLANCHNIC BLOOD VOLUME

At rest the splanchnic organs serve as a repository of some noncirculating blood. Exercise and hemorrhage mobilize this stored blood from its reservoirs, located mainly in the microscopic veins of the spleen and liver. The result is a reduction in splanchnic blood volume, as the expelled blood courses out of the splanchnic vessels, through the hepatic veins, and into the inferior vena cava. The mobilized blood increases the venous return to the heart, thereby augmenting the cardiac output, as a part of the overall cardiovascular response to exercise or hemorrhage. Still other circulatory disorders may increase the volume of blood in the splanchnic region.

Both passive and active factors influence splanchnic blood volume. Passive forces include the outflow pressure in the hepatic veins, the capacitance of storage sites in the venules of the splanchnic organs, and the rate of inflow of blood into these organs from the celiac and mesenteric arteries. Active forces include the tone of arterial and venous smooth muscle, which are mediated primarily by the splanchnic sympathetic nerves.

During exercise or hemorrhage, sympathetic nervous activity increases, and norepinephrine is released close to α-adrenergic receptors on the venular smooth muscle of splanchnic organs. Active contraction of these muscular structures expels much of the blood volume of the spleen and liver into the inferior vena cava, thereby contributing up to a liter of blood to the circulating blood volume. Norepinephrine also constricts splanchnic arterial smooth muscle, which decreases blood flow into the splanchnic organs and further reduces their blood volume. These organs are spared from hypoxic damage, at least for a time, because their cells extract a larger proportion of available oxygen from the blood whose flow has been reduced. Another stimulus that causes reduced splanchnic blood flow in the foregoing manner is the application of heat to the mucosa of the stomach, which would occur with the drinking of hot coffee or soup.

The blood volume of the liver and spleen rises when central venous pressure is elevated. A chronic elevation occurs during congestive cardiac failure because the heart is unable to pump the venous return in an efficient manner. This central obstruction to venous flow raises pressures in the vena cavae, hepatic veins, and portal vein. One result is a passive increase in the blood volume of the liver and spleen, sufficient to cause their enlargement. The findings of an enlarged liver and spleen by the physician during the physical examination of the patient's abdomen are important evidence in diagnosing congestive cardiac failure.

RESPONSE TO A MEAL

The major physiological challenge to the splanchnic circulation becomes evident with the consumption, digestion, and absorption of a meal. The alimentary tract is activated dramatically from near dormancy to maximal function by the sight, smell, taste, and ingestion of food. Within a matter of minutes the digestive system undergoes full stimulation of its main functions, which include: exocrine secretion of saliva, gastric and pancreatic juices, bile, and intestinal fluid; propulsive and churning motions of the pharynx, esophagus, stomach, gall bladder, and gut; synthesis and release of digestive enzymes; endocrine secretion of peptide hormones; active and passive transport of digested nutrients and fluids across the intestinal epithelium; extrinsic and intrinsic neuronal excitation in each organ; and intestinal mucosal metabolism of some nutrients (e.g., resynthesis of triglycerides and catabolism of glucose). Arousal of the digestive system heightens its need for energy in the form of an increased delivery of blood and oxygen to support the vital work of incorporating food into the body.

Central nervous, local metabolic, and local nervous mechanisms interact to mediate the hyperemic response to a meal. The reader is referred to Fig. 13-3 and the discussion of this diagram as background for the following explanation about the postprandial hyperemia.

The central nervous response to hunger and to food involves autonomic nerves. Central excitation of parasympathetics stimulates exocrine secretion and motor activity in the hollow organs of the gastrointestinal tract, which increases their metabolic activity. As will be described below, metabolic activation of cells leads to increased blood flow. Vagal excitation also initiates release of gastrointestinal hormones, which further stimulate secretion and motility of the hollow viscera. Lastly, extrinsic parasympathetic nerves synapse with intrinsic gastrointestinal nerves in the wall of the hollow organs, thereby triggering local nervous stimulation of secretion and motility and vasodilation of arterioles. Central nervous excitation of the sympathetic nervous system causes an increase in cardiac output, which makes more blood available to the splanchnic viscera.

The local metabolic mechanism that evokes an increase in blood flow involves increased oxygen consumption by activated cells leading to a decrease in Po_2. The latter effect relaxes vascular smooth muscle, prompting vasodilation and an increase in blood flow to the activated cells. Similarly, as cells are activated, vasodilator metabolites accumulate in higher concentrations and further relax vascular smooth muscle. Examples of such dilator metabolites include adenosine, prostacyclin, histamine, and bradykinin. Relaxation of arteriolar smooth muscle causes increased inflow of blood into the region in which cells are metabolically more active. Relaxation of the smooth muscle of precapillary sphincters opens up a larger population of capillaries to be perfused with blood and magnifies the surface area for exchange of oxygen and nutrients from blood to cells.

The need for oxygen to support some of the functions surrounding alimentation can be enormous for certain cells. For example, it has been estimated that the maximally secreting oxyntic gland region of the gastric mucosa consumes more oxygen per gram of tissue than any other tissue in the body under any conditions. Another example of the appetite for oxygen in cells that are involved in the processing of ingested nutrients can be observed during active cotransport of sodium and glucose across epithelial cells of the intestinal villi. With local usage of oxygen to support the needs of active transport and with the generation of vasodilator metabolites there is an increase in blood flow and an opening of more capillaries to permit increased surface area for movement of oxygen into metabolizing cells. The result is an increased extraction of oxygen from each milliliter of blood perfusing the intestinal mucosa. Hence the increase in oxygen consumption of the absorbing gut is proportionally greater than the increase in blood flow, because oxygen consumption is the product of blood flow times oxygen extraction.

The third mechanism leading to an increase in blood flow in the digestive system involves the intrinsic nerves. These nerves differ in terms of their neurotransmitter substances. Some of these nerves release a classical transmitter (i.e., acetylcholine or catecholamines). Other intrinsic nerves of the gut release purines, amines, or a variety of peptides. Some of the released peptides are identical with or closely related to gastrointestinal hormones, which are released from endocrine cells in the gastrointestinal mucosa or pancreas (e.g., CCK or VIP). Other peptides are unique neurotransmitter agents (e.g., substance P). These enteric transmitters are released near exocrine secretory cells or smooth muscle cells in the wall of the gut, where they can influence secretion, motility, and blood flow. Thus, for example, when ingested lipid is solubilized into micellar form in the intestinal lumen by bile acids preparatory to the diffusion of the micelles into epithelial cells, there is a sizeable increase in mucosal blood flow in the segment of gut in which the micelles have formed. The micelles excite local afferent C fibers in the wall of the gut, which transmit the neural message to nerve endings on the smooth muscle of mucosal arterioles. VIP is released and relaxes the smooth muscle to cause vasodilation and an increase in local blood flow.

The complex control of blood flow to the digestive organs at mealtimes assures the continuing availability of blood and oxygen to support the variety of digestive processes that occur over the hour or so of increased activity in several different organs. Long after the initial excitement over eating has been satisfied and the central nervous system is no longer stimulating an increased splanchnic blood flow, the gut and liver still have an enhanced blood supply because of local metabolic and intrinsic neural mechanisms.

SUGGESTED REFERENCES

Donald DE: Splanchnic circulation. In Sheperd JT, editor: Handbook of physiology: the cardiovascular system, Washington, DC, 1983, vol 3, American Physiological Society.

Granger DN, Kvietys PR, Perry MA, and Barrowman JA: The microcirculation and intestinal transport. In Johnson LR, editor: Physiology of the gastrointestinal tract, ed 2, New York, 1987, Raven Press.

Lundgren O: Microcirculation of the gastrointestinal tract and pancreas. In Renkin EM and Michel CC, editors: Handbook of physiology: the cardiovascular system, Washington, DC, 1984, vol 4, American Physiological Society.

Parks DA and Jacobson ED: Mesenteric circulation. In Johnson LR, editor: Physiology of the gastrointestinal tract, ed 2, New York, 1987, Raven Press.

Index

M

N